Understanding
Indigestion and Ulcers

Professor C.J. Hawkey and Dr N.J.D. Wight

Published by Family Doctor Publications Limited
in association with the British Medical Association

IMPORTANT
This book is intended not as a substitute for personal
medical advice but as a supplement to that advice for
the patient who wishes to understand more about his
or her condition.

Before taking any form of treatment
YOU SHOULD ALWAYS CONSULT YOUR MEDICAL
PRACTITIONER.

In particular (without limit) you should note that
advances in medical science occur rapidly and some
information about drugs and treatment contained in this
booklet may very soon be out of date.

ISBN-13: 978-1-903474-46-4
ISBN-10: 1-903474-46-9

Contents

About the authors

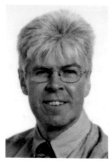

Professor C.J. Hawkey is Professor of Gastroenterology at Nottingham University and founding chairman of the Nottingham Gut Group. He was educated in Oxford and trained at the Middlesex Hospital. He has worked in many hospitals in England treating and researching this therapeutic area.

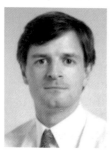

Dr N.J.D. Wight is a specialist registrar in Gastroenterology at the Queen's Medical Centre in Nottingham. His research interests include the interactions between *Helicobacter pylori* and non-steroidal anti-inflammatory drugs in the causation of peptic ulcers.

Introduction

A very common symptom

Virtually everyone has had indigestion at some time, and for most people it's simply a minor nuisance. More often than not, it happens when you've overindulged in food or alcohol or eaten something that doesn't agree with you, and it lasts for only a relatively short time.

In these situations, you can either wait for the symptoms to subside or treat yourself with a remedy from the pharmacist without needing to see a doctor.

For some people, however, the symptoms can be persistent and so severe that they interfere with everyday life. They may be caused by some undiagnosed problem within the digestive system that needs to be properly identified and, if necessary, treated by a doctor.

This book will help you distinguish between minor symptoms that you can safely treat yourself with the advice of a pharmacist and those that need further investigation.

The word 'indigestion' means different things to different people, but mostly it is used to describe discomfort in the central upper abdomen related in some way to eating or swallowing. Other common symptoms include:

- pain in the chest or abdomen

- a burning sensation in the chest (heartburn) often linked with food or liquid coming up into the throat or the back of the mouth (known medically as gastro-oesophageal reflux)

- belching or burping gas or wind into the mouth.

Treating indigestion

If you get such symptoms only occasionally, you should ask your pharmacist about over-the-counter treatments, which can be used safely to treat the odd bout of indigestion. You should also read the section in this book on lifestyle changes (see page 16) and make any necessary changes to reduce your chances of further attacks. Simple measures like these will usually be all that is needed to solve your problem, but in certain circumstances it is best to see your GP:

- If you have difficulty swallowing, unintentional weight loss, abdominal swelling, persistent vomiting or vomiting blood, you should make an urgent appointment to see your GP.

- If you have indigestion and are taking certain types of drugs, either prescribed or bought from the chemist, you should make a routine appointment to see your GP (the types of drugs that may cause indigestion are described in detail on pages 72–4).

- If your indigestion does not get better with simple over-the-counter remedies, you should make a routine appointment to see your GP.

Whether or not to see your GP is discussed in detail on pages 13–15. Remember, if self-help doesn't work, or if you are worried, it is always best to see your GP.

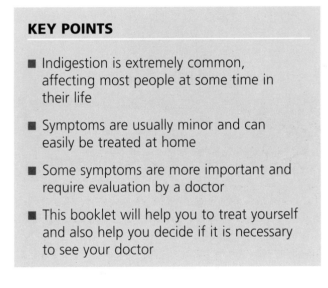

KEY POINTS

■ Indigestion is extremely common, affecting most people at some time in their life

■ Symptoms are usually minor and can easily be treated at home

■ Some symptoms are more important and require evaluation by a doctor

■ This booklet will help you to treat yourself and also help you decide if it is necessary to see your doctor

Normal digestion

How the digestive system works

Many people sometimes have only a vague idea of the size, shape, position and function of the stomach and other digestive organs. This section of the book gives a brief outline of the normal process of digestion and what each of the main parts of the digestive system does. If this is all familiar to you, just skip this account and move straight on to page 10, where the main types of indigestion are described.

To extract nutrients from the food that we eat we need to digest it. First the food has to be changed into a liquid or semi-liquid form. Then, complex substances such as fats and proteins have to be broken down into smaller chemical units that can be absorbed through the walls of the intestine into the bloodstream.

The mouth

The process of digestion begins in your mouth, where the teeth and tongue chop large pieces of food into smaller ones. The salivary glands release saliva into the mouth to mix with the food. Saliva makes it easier to

The structure of the mouth

The tongue, teeth and saliva work together to start the process of digestion. There are three pairs of salivary glands that aid the tasting, chewing and swallowing of food.

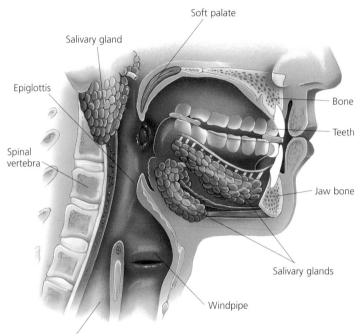

Soft palate

Salivary gland

Epiglottis

Bone

Teeth

Spinal vertebra

Jaw bone

Salivary glands

Windpipe

Oesophagus

move food round your mouth to chew it, and it also contains an enzyme called salivary amylase that starts to digest carbohydrates such as sugars and starches. It is slightly acid and, when you're not actually eating, it goes on being produced and helps to keep your mouth and teeth clean and stop plaque developing on your teeth. People who have conditions in which salivary production is reduced often experience a dry mouth, difficulty swallowing and increased tooth decay.

The stomach and intestines

Once the food is chewed and softened in the mouth, the tongue pushes it to the back of the throat, where muscles propel it down the oesophagus (or gullet). The food passes from the oesophagus into the stomach through a muscular one-way valve, the lower oesophageal sphincter, which prevents the contents of the stomach from being forced back into the chest when the stomach contracts or when you lie flat.

Functions of the stomach

The stomach is a muscular J-shaped sac that forms the widest part of the digestive tract. It has three main functions in the digestive process:

1. It acts as a storage container, so that within a few minutes we can swallow all the food needed for many hours.

2. It plays a large part in the physical and chemical processes of digestion. Food in the stomach is churned and crushed, although you notice this only when the activity is excessive because your stomach does not contain the same number of sensory nerves as other parts of the body, such as the skin. Glands within the stomach lining produce a powerful acid and enzymes that help break down the constituents of food into simpler chemical compounds. The walls of the stomach are normally protected against acid attack by a layer of protective mucus, but, if this is reduced or damaged, it may lead to ulcer formation. The oesophagus doesn't have this protective lining and so is more easily damaged by acid.

The major abdominal organs and digestion

Ingested food passes down the oesophagus and into the stomach, where it is churned and mixed thoroughly with digestive juices secreted by the stomach lining. Further digestive enzymes are added to the food in the duodenum.

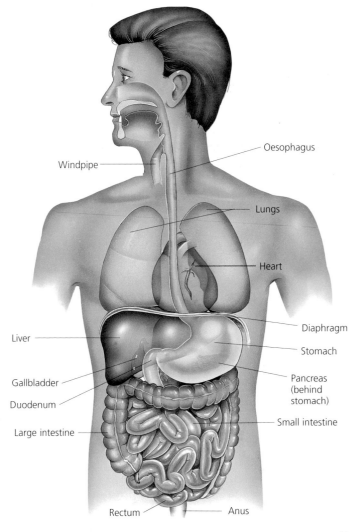

- Windpipe
- Oesophagus
- Lungs
- Heart
- Diaphragm
- Liver
- Stomach
- Gallbladder
- Pancreas (behind stomach)
- Duodenum
- Small intestine
- Large intestine
- Rectum
- Anus

Section through stomach wall

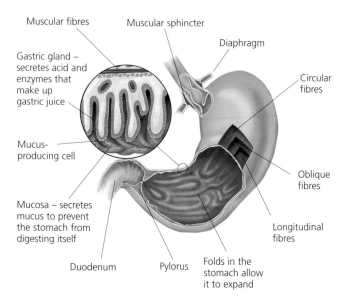

Muscular fibres

Muscular sphincter

Diaphragm

Gastric gland –
secretes acid and
enzymes that
make up
gastric juice

Circular
fibres

Mucus-
producing cell

Oblique
fibres

Mucosa – secretes
mucus to prevent
the stomach from
digesting itself

Longitudinal
fibres

Duodenum

Pylorus

Folds in the
stomach allow
it to expand

3. Food may stay in the stomach for several hours,
during which time the acid will destroy most of
the bacteria and other micro-organisms that may
have contaminated it. Very little is absorbed
directly into the bloodstream through the
stomach walls, apart from a few substances such
as alcohol and aspirin.

When the stomach has done its work the liquidised
food is then pushed onwards through another valve,
the pylorus, into the duodenum – the first few inches
of the small intestine. Here further chemicals are added
to neutralise the stomach acid, together with enzymes
from the pancreas to help digest carbohydrates, fats
and proteins, and bile from the liver to help digest fats.

The swallowing process

To allow you to swallow food safely, two involuntary events occur: the soft palate rises to close off the nasal cavity and the epiglottis tilts to seal the windpipe.

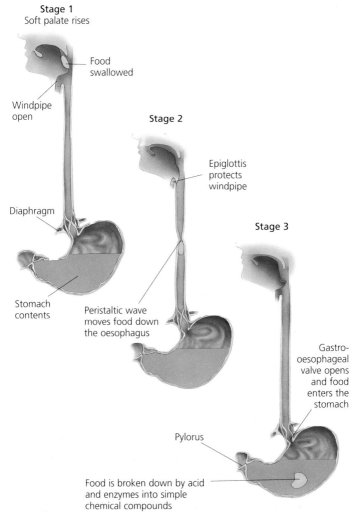

Stage 1
Soft palate rises

Food swallowed

Windpipe open

Diaphragm

Stomach contents

Stage 2

Epiglottis protects windpipe

Peristaltic wave moves food down the oesophagus

Stage 3

Gastro-oesophageal valve opens and food enters the stomach

Pylorus

Food is broken down by acid and enzymes into simple chemical compounds

The digested food then passes into the remaining 20 feet (six metres) of small intestine, so called because, although it is long, its diameter is smaller than that of the large intestine. The chemical breakdown is completed in the small intestine and the chemical constituents of the meal are absorbed into the blood and lymphatic vessels.

The main tasks of the large intestine are to reabsorb the water that is used in digestion and to eliminate the undigested food and fibre.

What can go wrong?

Almost everyone experiences occasional attacks of indigestion, which are usually quite brief. We may feel blown out or distended after a large meal, and get some relief when we bring up wind. Most of the wind that we bring up is a result of swallowing air as we eat, but some is produced by a chemical reaction in the stomach or from carbonated, fizzy drinks. The solutions are to eat less, eat more slowly and go easy with fizzy drinks. You may have discovered for yourself that certain foods – fried onions, for example – give you an uncomfortable sensation in the upper abdomen that lasts for only an hour or so. Again the answer is obvious: don't eat those foods, or avoid them where possible.

Causes of indigestion

More persistent indigestion is usually linked with the acid produced by the stomach. If the valve at the lower end of the oesophagus becomes weak or defective, the acid juices in the stomach may be pushed back upwards into the oesophagus, causing a burning sensation (heartburn). This is often troublesome at night, when you lie flat. The underlying condition is called gastro-oesophageal reflux and is described in more detail on pages 43–60.

Stomach acid may also cause problems if it attacks the lining of the stomach itself, known as peptic ulcer disease, described in detail later (see page 61). Our understanding of peptic ulcer disease has changed greatly in recent years, thanks to the discovery of an infective agent called *Helicobacter pylori* – you'll find out more about this later (see page 64).

The third common cause of indigestion, called non-ulcer dyspepsia, is something of a puzzle. This is the diagnosis given to people who have persistent symptoms of indigestion but in whom the tests for gastro-oesophageal reflux and stomach ulcers are normal. Dyspepsia is actually just the medical name for indigestion. Some people with this type of indigestion are eventually found to have a disorder affecting another part of the digestive system, such as gallstones or the irritable bowel syndrome. In others, the pain is found to be caused by some disorder of the lower ribs and muscles of the abdominal wall. Most people with non-ulcer dyspepsia, however, seem to have sensitive stomachs that cause symptoms at times of emotional stress. The condition is described in greater detail on pages 87–92.

Very occasionally, indigestion may be the first symptom of a more serious condition such as stomach cancer. Stomach cancer is becoming less common than in the past and it occurs far less frequently than peptic ulcer disease or gastro-oesophageal reflux. It is described in greater detail on pages 93–9.

KEY POINTS

■ During the normal digestion process, food is broken down so that it can be absorbed into the body

■ The stomach produces acid and pepsin to help in this process

■ If the lining of the stomach is weakened, or if acid production is altered, then indigestion can occur

Do you need to see your doctor?

Assessing the seriousness of your condition

Probably three of every four people who suffer from indigestion never seek medical advice: they relieve their symptoms by a few changes to their lifestyle and by taking over-the-counter treatments, such as antacids or acid-blocking drugs, bought from the chemist every now and then.

One of the aims of this book is to help you decide whether and when to consult your doctor. You should make an appointment if any of the three following situations applies to you.

Sinister symptoms

See your GP without delay if you have any symptoms of the kind that doctors call 'sinister', by which they mean symptoms that might be caused by a serious disease such as stomach cancer. Early diagnosis and treatment give the best chance of a cure, so get prompt medical advice if you have any of the following symptoms:

- unintentional weight loss

- difficulty swallowing

- abdominal swelling

- persistent vomiting

- vomiting blood or material that looks like coffee grounds

- passing altered blood in the motions (this makes your stools look like tar).

Medicine interactions
Make a routine appointment to see your GP if you develop indigestion while taking any of the following drugs or tablets:

- certain blood pressure drugs known as calcium channel antagonists (nifedipine, amlodipine and verapamil are examples)

- nitrate drugs for treatment of angina (such as isosorbide mononitrate)

- asthma drugs such as theophyllines

- bisphosphonate drugs used for the treatment of osteoporosis (alendronate and risedronate are examples)

- steroid tablets

- non-steroidal anti-inflammatory drugs such as ibuprofen, naproxen and diclofenac.

Prolonged indigestion
Make a routine appointment to see your GP if your indigestion does not go away despite the use of

over-the-counter medicines or if you need to take these medicines for a prolonged period of time.

Your doctor may need to arrange various tests and investigations before beginning treatment – this is covered on pages 28–41.

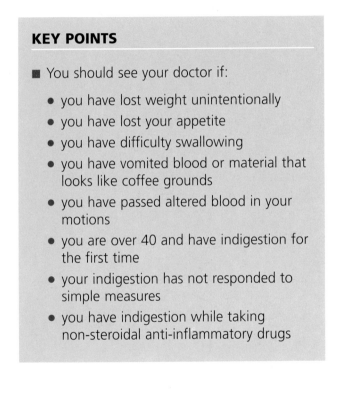

KEY POINTS

■ You should see your doctor if:

- you have lost weight unintentionally
- you have lost your appetite
- you have difficulty swallowing
- you have vomited blood or material that looks like coffee grounds
- you have passed altered blood in your motions
- you are over 40 and have indigestion for the first time
- your indigestion has not responded to simple measures
- you have indigestion while taking non-steroidal anti-inflammatory drugs

Treating indigestion yourself

What you can do

Symptoms of indigestion are so common that we tend to think of them as something quite minor, which we can treat ourselves with medicines bought over the counter at the chemist. The range of remedies on offer is huge and they sell in great quantities. However, it is worth bearing in mind that symptoms mean that something is going wrong somewhere in the digestive system and, if you have anything more than the occasional mild attack, it is necessary to seek out and treat the cause rather than just dealing with the symptoms themselves. If simple self-help measures don't solve the problem, you should make an appointment to see your GP.

Changing your lifestyle

If you have recently had one or two attacks of mild indigestion it is worth trying to make some changes in your lifestyle that will be kinder to your stomach. It is also important to improve your health in general.

Lifestyle changes that can help you avoid indigestion include:

- If you smoke you should stop.

- Try to lose weight and increase the amount of exercise you take – instead of taking the bus or driving you should walk or cycle and take the stairs not the lift.

- Do not drink too much alcohol. Men should not take more than 24 units of alcohol a week (one unit is equal to half a pint of beer or lager, a glass of wine or a measure of spirits ['short']). Women should not take more than 14 units of alcohol a week.

- Eat a healthier diet. Cut down on the amount of fatty foods you eat including fried food, butter, cheese, crisps and red meat. Instead, eat more fruit, grilled chicken or fish and try boiled potatoes instead of chips.

- Increase the amount of fibre in your diet. Fibre is found in fruit and vegetables and in high-fibre breakfast cereals and whole-grain bread.

- Avoid hot spices, salt and vinegar and certain salads (onions and tomatoes) as these often make heartburn worse.

- Decrease your caffeine intake by reducing the amount of tea and coffee you have. Try decaffeinated coffee and, if you take fizzy drinks, try decaffeinated ones.

- Don't eat a large meal just before you go to bed; allow a few hours for your food to digest before lying down.

- Stomachs like routine and work better when you eat three or four meals at the same times each day.

- Anxiety and stress affect the way the stomach muscles work so try to take some time in the day to relax on your own for a short while.

Medicines can cause indigestion

Indigestion can be made worse or even be caused by treatment with medicines such as aspirin and other non-steroidal anti-inflammatory drugs taken for arthritis and other painful disorders. These drugs reduce inflammation by decreasing the body's production of chemicals called prostaglandins. As well as causing inflammation in the joints, however, these chemicals also help the stomach protect itself against acid. This is why indigestion and ulcers are a common side effect of these types of drugs. For more detail on this, see pages 72–4.

You may find that taking paracetamol, which does not irritate the stomach, instead of aspirin may relieve your indigestion, but don't stop taking other anti-inflammatory drugs prescribed by your doctor without discussing it with him or her first.

Ask the pharmacist

Making changes to your lifestyle isn't always sufficient to get rid of your indigestion but, if you have no worrying symptoms (see page 2), it is reasonable to try treating your indigestion yourself for a couple of weeks. Making the right choice of over-the-counter medicine isn't easy, and the best person to advise you is the pharmacist. He or she will be able to recommend the right type of medication for your particular symptoms and will also know whether it is safe to take it at the same time as any other prescription medicines that you may be on. Ask about cost before making up your mind too – for example, some heavily advertised medications may be more expensive than identical products sold by pharmacy chains under their own brand names.

To help the pharmacist to help you, you will need to explain your symptoms and be able to say when you get them and so on. The checklist in the box below may be useful in getting the relevant facts sorted out in your mind before you go.

Over-the-counter remedies

There are several different types of indigestion remedy that you can buy over the counter without prescription.

What kind of pain or discomfort are you experiencing with your indigestion?

The pharmacist will need to know your symptoms to give you the best advice.

- When do you get the pain?
- What makes it worse?
- What makes it better?
- Have you lost weight recently?
- Do you have any other symptoms besides indigestion?
- What have you tried already?
- Are you or could you be pregnant?

Antacids

These are simple alkalis that neutralise stomach acid for a short period. Examples of simple alkalis are aluminium hydroxide, magnesium trisilicate and sodium bicarbonate. Generally, they have no harmful effects, although some people do have problems with their side effects on the bowels. Aluminium-containing antacids can cause constipation and magnesium-containing ones can cause diarrhoea. If you have other medical conditions or are taking other prescribed medicines, you should discuss these with your pharmacist

How antacids reduce stomach acidity

Antacids are simple alkalis, taken by mouth in a tablet or liquid form, that neutralise the acid in the stomach for a short period. They have relatively few side effects but can worsen certain medical conditions.

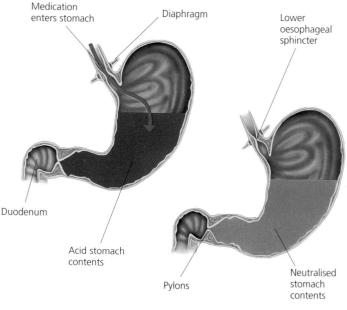

Medication enters stomach

Diaphragm

Lower oesophageal sphincter

Duodenum

Acid stomach contents

Pylons

Neutralised stomach contents

or your doctor before taking any of these over-the-counter medicines. This is especially important for anyone with heart disease, kidney disease or high blood pressure as many antacids contain salt (in the form of sodium bicarbonate), which can make these conditions worse. Some antacids (especially sodium bicarbonate) produce gas as they work and this can cause belching. Dimeticone is a chemical that is often added to antacids to help reduce flatulence.

Drugs that protect the stomach and oesophagus lining

These drugs form a protective lining around the stomach and oesophagus protecting against acid damage. They usually have several ingredients and often contain an antacid, but the main ingredient is alginate (made from seaweed), which floats on the stomach contents. If gastro-oesophageal reflux occurs (see page 43), the alginate soothes the lining of the oesophagus. Examples of alginate-containing drugs are Algicon, Gastrocote and Gaviscon. As these drugs all contain some antacid (sometimes containing salt) you should talk to your doctor or pharmacist before using them if you have other medical conditions or if you take other medicines.

Antispasmodics

These drugs act by reducing the tension in the muscle wall of the stomach. Examples of antispasmodics are alverine citrate and peppermint oil. Peppermint-containing chewing gum has a similar effect. These drugs are most effective if you suffer from a 'nervous stomach' or trapped wind. These drugs, being natural products, have no significant side effects.

Medicines that protect

Medicines that contain alginate are taken by mouth. They float on top of the stomach contents and, if acid reflux occurs, the alginate protects against acid damage by forming a protective lining around the oesophagus.

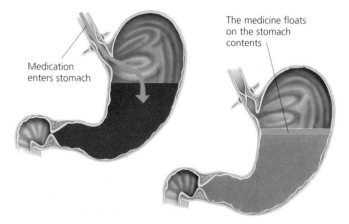

Medication enters stomach

The medicine floats on the stomach contents

Drugs that reduce stomach acid production

These drugs work by reducing the amount of acid produced by the stomach. They are very powerful and usually available only on prescription from your doctor. They are discussed in more detail later in the book.

Some acid-suppressing drugs, known medically as H_2-receptor antagonists, are, however, available over the counter, for example, cimetidine, famotidine and ranitidine. The doses that you can buy are lower than those normally prescribed by a doctor and they are only available in two-week packs. If your symptoms persist after two weeks of treatment you should see a doctor.

H_2-receptor antagonists have been in use for many years now and several hundred million patients have taken them without side effects. Nevertheless, a minority of people may develop side effects when

Acid-suppressing drugs

These are powerful drugs that should be used with caution and for limited periods of time.

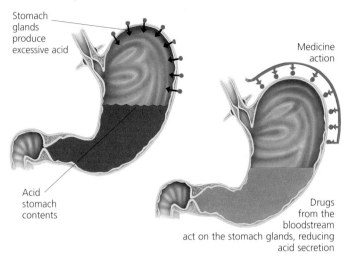

Stomach glands produce excessive acid

Acid stomach contents

Medicine action

Drugs from the bloodstream act on the stomach glands, reducing acid secretion

taking them, including drowsiness, headache, rash and confusion (especially in elderly people).

In particular, cimetidine can affect the way that other medicines are processed by the liver (especially warfarin, used to thin the blood, phenytoin, used in the treatment of epilepsy, and aminophylline, used in the treatment of chronic asthma). You should not take cimetidine if you are also taking one of these other drugs.

Which remedy is best?

The choice of over-the-counter remedies is vast and there is no real evidence that one is better than another. The best one is probably the one that you find most palatable and effective. They all taste different and some trial and error may be required. The best time to take your antacid is usually before the time that you would normally expect your symptoms to occur – soon after meals and before bedtime – but again trial and error is often required.

Indigestion remedies available from your pharmacist

Examples of the main types of indigestion remedies available from pharmacies are listed below.

Medicine class	Action	Proprietary or brand name
Antacids	Neutralise stomach acid	Aludrox tablets, Rennie, Setlers tablets, soda mint tablets
Drugs that protect the stomach and oesophagus lining	Line the stomach and oesophagus preventing acid damage	Algicon, Gastrocote, Gaviscon (these also contain antacid)
Anti-spasmodics	Reduce tension in the stomach wall muscles. Reduce bloatedness	Spasmonal, Colpermin, Mintec, peppermint chewing gum
H_2-receptor antagonists	Reduce stomach acid production	Tagamet, Pepcid, Boots Excess Acid Control, Zantac

KEY POINTS

■ People who smoke get more indigestion than people who don't

■ A lot of indigestion is brought on by eating the 'wrong' food, such as fatty food

■ Often improving the healthiness of your lifestyle will cure indigestion completely

■ A large number of indigestion remedies are available over the counter at the pharmacy

■ A pharmacist will be able to advise you which remedy is most suitable

What your doctor will do

Diagnosing the problem

If your indigestion does not clear up after two weeks with simple home treatment, it is sensible to ask your doctor's advice without further delay.

He or she will start off by asking a lot of questions about the exact symptoms that you have been experiencing, how long they have been troubling you, what brings them on, what relieves them, and so on. This will usually be followed by a physical examination to identify any tender places in your abdomen and to check on your general health.

Your family doctor may be confident that he or she can deal with your problem straight away, or you may be referred to a hospital clinic for further tests. In fact, most people with indigestion do not need further tests.

Your doctor will usually be able to make an accurate diagnosis based entirely on your symptoms and then offer advice or treatment. If the symptoms suggest gastro-oesophageal reflux then advice about lifestyle, with or without antacids, will usually be all

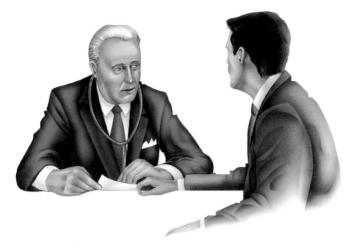

Your doctor will ask you detailed questions about any symptoms that you may be experiencing.

that you need. There are, however, three scenarios in which your doctor may feel that further investigation is warranted.

A suspected peptic ulcer

If your doctor suspects that your symptoms are caused by a peptic ulcer then you will be offered a test to see if you have the bacterium that causes ulcers. The bacterium is called *Helicobacter pylori* (see page 63).

Failure to respond to treatment

If you are one of the minority of people whose symptoms continue to be troublesome despite treatment, your doctor may arrange for you to have an endoscopy (passing a fibreoptic tube via the oesophagus into the stomach) to make sure that you don't have another condition that needs to be treated in a different way.

Sinister symptoms

This term is used to describe symptoms that almost always indicate significant underlying disease and warrant further investigation. The most important are indigestion associated with loss of appetite and weight, and difficulty swallowing. These symptoms always need urgent medical advice.

Further investigations may also be recommended if your symptoms have started recently and you are over 40 years old and the symptoms persist despite simple remedies. Stomach cancer is very unusual in younger patients, but it is always a possibility in patients with sinister symptoms or in older patients with any persistent symptoms.

Tests and investigations

Hospitals vary in the way that they organise tests requested by your GP: you may see one of the hospital doctors, or you may simply go for tests so that the results can then be sent to your own doctor who will decide what needs to be done next. There are various tests that you might need, but they are likely to include one or more of the following:

- Routine blood tests: these are simply to check for common abnormalities such as anaemia. Your doctor may take the opportunity of a blood test to check for other common diseases unrelated to your stomach.

- Endoscopy (see pages 29–35).

- Barium X-rays (see pages 35–7).

- Tests for *Helicobacter pylori* (*H. pylori*) infection (see pages 37–40). This type of investigation is different from the previous two tests in that it is not looking for anything abnormal within the oesophagus or the stomach but for the actual cause of the problem.

Endoscopy

An endoscope is an instrument that allows a doctor to look inside your body. There are endoscopes to examine joints (such as the knee), the lungs and the windpipe, the lower bowel and the bladder, as well as the oesophagus, stomach and duodenum. This section is concerned with the endoscopes used to look inside the oesophagus, the stomach and the duodenum.

The early endoscopes used lenses and mirrors, but 30 years ago these were replaced by fibreoptic instruments, which gave the operator a clear, direct view of the inside of the stomach.

Modern endoscopes are very advanced bits of technology (and thus extraordinarily expensive),

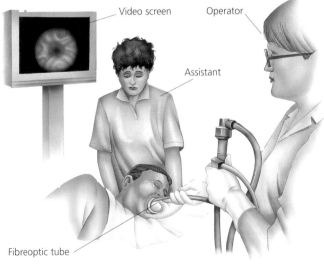

An endoscopy test.

consisting of a flexible piece of tubing, the tip of which can be controlled by the operator.

Older endoscopes have optical fibres along their length, but modern instruments actually have a small video camera in the tip and images are carried electronically direct to a video screen.

The instrument also has other channels for suctioning stomach juice, for blowing air to inflate the stomach, and for passing specialised forceps to take tiny biopsy specimens.

An endoscopy test (often called a gastroscopy or simply the telescope test) is now the most accurate and most useful way of investigating the different causes of indigestion. It is the best way of diagnosing peptic ulcers and stomach cancers, and can also be useful in diagnosing *H. pylori* infection.

As well as giving the operator a clear view of any abnormalities, it also allows him or her to take tissue samples (biopsies) if necessary, and can be used for treating other complications such as narrowing of the oesophagus.

Having an endoscopy test

Depending on your symptoms, your GP may refer you to the hospital clinic for a full assessment or just for the endoscopy itself – a system known as 'fast track' or 'open access' endoscopy.

Preparation and arrival at hospital

The procedure is usually carried out in a specialised unit within a hospital and takes only a few minutes. Endoscopy departments are extraordinarily busy places, however, and the check-in procedure before the test and booking out after the test may take an hour each.

It is usually best to set aside the whole morning or afternoon depending on the time of your appointment. Your stomach needs to be empty for a complete test. So, for a morning test you'll be told to eat or drink nothing after your evening meal on the previous day, and for an afternoon test to eat nothing after a light breakfast.

When you arrive at the department you will initially be directed to a waiting area with other patients and thence to an area where you can be 'clerked in' by either a doctor or a nurse.

The purpose of this is to explain the test and to answer your questions, but also to make sure that your general health is good enough, although it is very rare for anyone to be considered too ill to undergo the procedure. You will also be asked to sign a consent form. When it is your turn you will then be directed into the endoscopy room itself.

It is easy to be daunted by the numerous racks of equipment and machines in the endoscopy suite, but each has its own job to do and is individually straightforward.

The most important pieces are the endoscope itself and its accompanying operating equipment, a video screen where the pictures appear, and a machine for measuring your pulse and oxygen levels with a clip on your finger. This clever clip device works by shining a light through the soft tissue of your finger; changes in the amount of light absorbed show how 'red' your blood is and thus how much oxygen it is carrying.

The test itself
As well as the endoscopist, there will also be a nurse to look after you and another member of staff to assist the endoscopist. You will be asked to lie down on your

Anaesthesia during endoscopy

Having an endoscope passed down your throat can cause some discomfort so you may be offered a choice between two kinds of anaesthetic.

Some people feel that they will not be able to manage without some sedation, whereas others prefer to be wide awake and remain in control. Which option you choose depends on how you feel about the test.

Both methods have advantages and disadvantages and the final choice is usually left to the individual concerned, although different departments have different ways of working.

What are the choices?

1. Throat spray

This is the simplest option. Before inserting the endoscope, the endoscopist or assistant sprays some local anaesthetic solution into the back of your throat, making it numb. You then lie comfortably on your side and remain wide awake throughout the test. The main advantage of having only the throat spray is that you remain in complete control throughout the procedure. Also, because you are not sedated, you may well be able to discuss the results of the test straightaway and be able to drive yourself home or back to work afterwards. The disadvantage of the throat spray is that, because there is no sedative effect, anyone who is very anxious may be unable to swallow the endoscope and complete the test. The throat spray affects swallowing for up to 30 minutes after use, so you

Anaesthesia during endoscopy (contd)

are advised not to eat or drink until sensation has completely returned to normal, to prevent food and liquids being inhaled or 'going down the wrong way'.

2. Intravenous sedation

This method is a little more time-consuming and requires the endoscopist to place a temporary needle in the back of your hand or arm before giving a sedative injection. It doesn't render you unconscious (unlike a general anaesthetic) but makes you feel much more relaxed and comfortable. You are still able to hear and to swallow when asked to do so. The main advantage of intravenous sedation is that it makes the test easier to cope with if you are anxious and you may not remember anything about it afterwards. The main disadvantage is that you may become disoriented and the effects of sedation take several hours to wear off completely. This means that you will need someone else to drive you home and you will not be able to return to work the same day. In fact, it's always a good idea to take someone with you when having an endoscopy, even if you plan to have throat spray rather than sedation, in case you change your mind at the last minute.

Another disadvantage of sedation is that you may not be able to get any results on the day of the test because of the effects on your memory. Endoscopy itself does not interfere with breathing in any way, but intravenous sedation can suppress breathing so it may not be suitable if you have heart or lung disease. Some departments also give a throat spray to some patients in addition to sedation.

left side and will be made comfortable. You may be given a sedative injection or have some throat spray depending on which you prefer (see box on pages 32–3).

The nurse will then place the monitoring clip on your finger and may give you some oxygen (usually with a sponge-tipped tube up your nose) before placing a small mouth guard between your teeth. This protects both your teeth from the endoscope and the endoscope from your teeth.

When ready the endoscopist will place the tip of the endoscope over your tongue and into your throat. You will then be asked to swallow and, as you do so, the oesophagus will open up allowing the endoscope to pass down into your stomach.

The nurse looking after you during the test will constantly remove saliva from your mouth with a sucker, much like that used by dentists, which helps reduce the risk of you inhaling any fluid. You will be able to swallow with the tube in your throat, but fluid can collect in your mouth because the tube holds open the oesophagus, allowing liquid to reflux up from your stomach.

Once the endoscope is in position the test takes only a few minutes, during which time air is blown into the stomach so that a good view can be obtained. Depending on the findings, the endoscopist may take some biopsies (tissue samples), which is an entirely painless process.

When the examination is complete the endoscope is withdrawn and you are taken back to the 'recovery' area. During the test the main symptoms that you can expect are pressure within the throat and occasionally some tummy discomfort and belching because of the air that is introduced. As the scope is passed into your throat you may retch once or twice, which is a normal reaction and usually minor. Once you have completely recovered after the test you can go home.

Is endoscopy safe?

Endoscopy departments are very busy places and every member of staff that you meet there will be an expert with a lot of experience. Endoscopy is an extremely safe procedure and serious complications of a simple diagnostic test are virtually unheard of. Very rarely, however, the oesophagus may tear as the endoscope is being inserted, but this usually only happens in patients with previously undiagnosed abnormalities of the upper oesophagus. In any case, the risk is probably less than one per 10,000 procedures.

Other less serious complications relate to intravenous sedation: if liquid is inhaled it may cause a chest infection, but this is very rare during a simple diagnostic test and is more likely to occur in frail and elderly people.

Barium X-rays

Barium X-rays are used far less nowadays than in the past, because in most cases an endoscopy examination will give all the information needed. However, some GPs may not have access to a hospital department offering an endoscopy service and so may refer their patients for a barium X-ray instead.

In any case, this may be a better option for some individuals, especially if the problem is in the oesophagus, as the test shows up its structure and any muscle spasm will be visible.

A barium 'swallow' X-ray

Barium is drunk in a soluton into the patient's empty stomach.
Barium is opaque to X-rays, so it shows up on film revealing any
diseases or abnormalities of the large intestine.

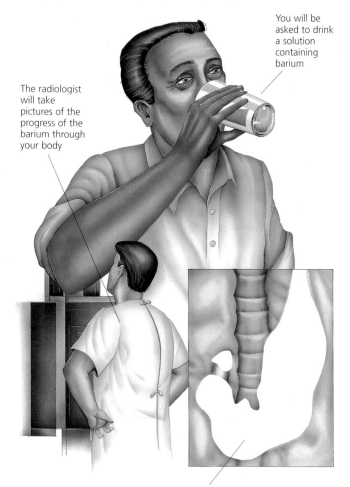

You will be
asked to drink
a solution
containing
barium

The radiologist
will take
pictures of the
progress of the
barium through
your body

Radiograph or X-ray
of a normal stomach
after a barium meal

Why is barium useful?

Ordinary X-ray examinations of the kind used to assess broken bones give poor images of the internal organs. If, however, some barium sulphate is swallowed before the X-rays are taken it outlines the shape of the oesophagus and stomach. Barium is a heavy metal that is totally impenetrable by X-rays and so shows up on films and screens as opaque shadows. Barium sulphate is tasteless and causes no discomfort when you swallow it.

Taking the test

Barium X-ray examinations are generally carried out in the outpatient department and you don't need an anaesthetic. The radiologist uses a fluorescent screen to watch the progress of the barium after you have swallowed it, and he or she will take pictures from time to time to provide a permanent record.

The whole examination usually takes about 20 to 30 minutes. The barium is eventually passed out in the faeces; it sometimes causes constipation, so you should eat a high-fibre diet for a day or two after the test.

Tests for *Helicobacter pylori*

If you are thought likely to be suffering from peptic ulcer disease, tests will be needed to determine whether your stomach is infected with *Helicobacter pylori*. This infection has an important role in causing ulcers, which is explained on page 64. There are four ways of testing for *H. pylori*:

1. Examining a tissue sample from the stomach lining (a biopsy)

2. A breath test

3. A blood test

4. A stool test.

Tissue tests

These require a tiny specimen of the stomach lining, called a biopsy, which is taken during an endoscopy. The specimen is placed in a special solution (either liquid or gel), which changes colour if *H. pylori* is present; this is called a urease test. *H. pylori* organisms secrete a protein chemical called urease, which converts urea (a substance present in the bloodstream and in urine produced by the breakdown of protein) to ammonia.

The diagnostic solutions contain urea and an alkali indicator. If *H. pylori* is present within the biopsy placed in the test solution then the urea is converted into ammonia, which causes the alkali indicator to change colour, thus producing a positive test. Depending on which test solution is used, the result takes from a few minutes to 24 hours to become available.

In addition to the urease test, the biopsy specimen can also be sent to the pathology department to be looked at under a microscope. Not only can the microscopic *H. pylori* themselves be seen in this way, but so can the associated microscopic stomach inflammation called gastritis.

The main advantage of these tests is that they are the most accurate available and confirm whether or not active *H. pylori* is present at the time of the test. In addition, while performing the endoscopy, the doctor can see if there is any evidence of a peptic ulcer, suggesting that *H. pylori* should be eradicated.

The disadvantage of tissue testing is that it requires an endoscopy, but looking for *H. pylori* is rarely the only reason for doing such an investigation, so it makes sense to do a biopsy at the same time anyway.

In common with some other *H. pylori* tests, the results can be incorrectly interpreted if you are taking a type of medication called proton pump inhibitor therapy (such as omeprazole, lansoprazole or pantoprazole, see page 52), which suppresses the bacterium without actually killing it.

Breath test

Like the tissue test, the urea breath test makes use of the fact that *H. pylori* secretes urease, which converts urea into ammonia, producing carbon dioxide as it does so. You are asked to eat nothing for 12 hours before a breath test and are then given a drink containing urea, to which a tiny amount of perfectly safe radiation has been added. Thirty minutes later, a small breath sample is collected. If *H. pylori* is present in your stomach the urea is converted into ammonia and carbon dioxide, which is then absorbed and excreted in your breath, along with a tiny amount of radioactivity. This can then be measured with a special machine in the hospital laboratory.

The advantage of the breath test is that it is very straightforward and takes a very short amount of time. Like the biopsy urease test, it is very accurate and confirms that you have active *H. pylori* infection at the time of the test. This also means that, if necessary, the breath test can be performed repeatedly to check whether the bacterium has been eradicated after treatment.

The disadvantage of the test, like some other *H. pylori* tests, is that the result may be inaccurate if you are taking proton pump inhibitor medication (see page 52). Also, the result is not usually available for several days because of the measuring equipment used.

Antibody blood test

As with other infections, *H. pylori* infection triggers the production of specific antibodies in your blood. These can be looked for with a simple blood test and their presence confirms *H. pylori* infection. However, once your body has produced these antibodies they may persist for many years, even after the infection has been eradicated.

For this reason, the blood test is useful for diagnosing infection only in a person who has never had *H. pylori* treatment. The real advantage of the blood test is that it is very quick and is usually available in the GP's surgery. Unlike the other tests for *H. pylori*, the blood test is not influenced by any drugs that you may be taking.

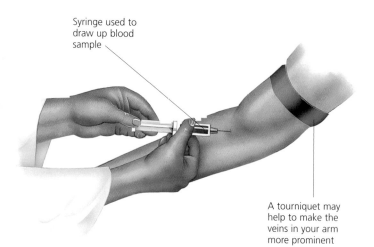

Syringe used to draw up blood sample

A tourniquet may help to make the veins in your arm more prominent

Taking a blood sample.

Stool test

A new test involves collection of a sample of your stool, which is tested to detect evidence of *H. pylori* in the stomach.

Test and treat

If your GP suspects a peptic ulcer you will be offered one of the tests for *Helicobacter pylori* described above. If the test is positive you will be given treatment for the infection. If it is negative then your GP will review your symptoms.

KEY POINTS

- Your doctor will ask about your symptoms and examine you

- Often the cause of indigestion is straightforward and your doctor can offer you treatment immediately

- If your doctor suspects a peptic ulcer or something more serious, then special tests will be arranged

- The most usual test is to look into the stomach with a telescope – an endoscopy test

- Other tests that are sometimes used are blood tests, barium X-rays and tests for *Helicobacter pylori* infecton

Heartburn

Gastro-oesophageal reflux

Gastro-oesophageal reflux is the medical name for what most of us refer to as heartburn, although it can also cause other symptoms besides the burning pain in the centre of your chest. It is the most common cause of indigestion and will affect most people at some stage in their lives.

What are the symptoms?

The symptoms of heartburn are usually relatively trivial, but they are often long-standing and can become quite disabling. The most common symptom produced by gastro-oesophageal reflux is the burning sensation that can radiate into the throat. It often comes and goes and can be brought on by certain foods, by stooping, or by lying flat in bed at night. Sometimes it is associated with difficulty swallowing or with painful swallowing. Occasionally gastro-oesophageal reflux may cause regurgitation of food into the mouth and a feeling of nausea.

How does gastro-oesophageal reflux occur?

This symptom occurs when the acidic stomach contents leak out of the stomach into the oesophagus, causing the symptoms that we know as heartburn. This happens when the valve at the top of the stomach fails to remain tightly closed.

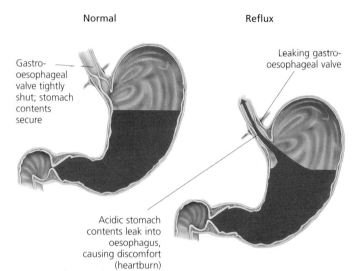

Normal   Reflux

Gastro-oesophageal valve tightly shut; stomach contents secure

Leaking gastro-oesophageal valve

Acidic stomach contents leak into oesophagus, causing discomfort (heartburn)

How is it treated?

Often, a change in lifestyle is all that is required for most people, but there are also a number of useful antacid treatments available from the chemist (see page 24), and for more severe cases there are a number of highly effective drugs now available on prescription.

Heartburn or angina?

It is important to point out that, in the vast majority of cases, gastro-oesophageal reflux is not serious and doesn't mean you have or are likely to develop, another illness such as cancer. However, it is important to distinguish heartburn from another common cause of central chest pain, especially in men or women over 50, namely angina.

Angina pain is usually brought on by exertion, such as brisk walking uphill, and is quickly relieved by rest, unlike reflux, so it is usually not difficult to tell one from the other. If you have pain that you think might be angina, you should consult your doctor without delay.

What causes gastro-oesophageal reflux?

As explained earlier (see page 6), the glands in the stomach produce a cocktail of hydrochloric acid and pepsin (an enzyme) to aid in the initial breakdown and subsequent digestion of food. In addition, this cocktail acts as a first step in destroying any bacteria present in food.

The stomach protects itself from the dangerous effects of the acid/pepsin mixture with a lining of special mucus. When the mixture leaves the stomach on its way into the intestine (the first part of which is called the duodenum), the acid is neutralised by alkaline juice from the pancreas.

The oesophagus (food-pipe) is rather sensitive to acid, but in normal circumstances this is not important because the junction between the stomach and oesophagus is held tightly closed by a valve (the gastro-oesophageal valve), thus preventing any of the stomach contents from passing back up the oesophagus. Occasionally, however, the gastro-oesophageal valve is not completely tight and so allows acid and pepsin back up into the oesophagus, causing the symptoms outlined on page 43.

The gastro-oesophageal valve has two components: the lower oesophageal sphincter muscle (the circular

Signs of a more serious condition

Although heartburn in itself is not normally serious, chest discomfort may sometimes be a sign that you have angina. You need to see your doctor without delay to find out what is causing your symptoms if:

- you develop pain in the centre of your chest or upper abdomen for the first time
- the pain changes in character or becomes more severe than usual
- the pain is brought on by exercise and goes away when you rest
- the pain radiates into your arms or neck
- you experience other symptoms as well as pain, including sweating, nausea, shortness of breath, faintness, passing out or palpitations.

Burping or wind can be caused by angina as well as by heartburn so it is of itself not a clue to the correct diagnosis.

muscle fibres that squeeze the passage shut) and the slit-like opening in the diaphragm muscle through which the oesophagus passes (the diaphragm hiatus).

Individually these two components are weak, but when working together they provide a tight junction. The function of this junction is very complex, and in the normal situation it is controlled by various reflexes. When we swallow, for example, the junction is required to relax at just the right time to allow food into the stomach, but when we are not swallowing the junction must remain tight to prevent gastro-oesophageal reflux.

Problems with the gastro-oesophageal valve

There are two main reasons why you may develop problems with your gastro-oesophageal valve. These may occur alone or together:

1. The sphincter muscle at the bottom of the oesophagus may relax too much.

2. You may develop a fault where the oesophagus passes through the diaphragm – a hiatus hernia.

Sphincter muscle problems

In some people there may be no obvious explanation why this muscle does not relax as it should, but factors that are known to play a part are:

- being overweight

- alcohol consumption

- smoking

- certain foodstuffs (fatty foods, onions and spicy foods, chocolate and acidic foods)

- occasionally prescribed drugs.

All of these are more likely to cause problems near bedtime, so that you are at increased risk of reflux when you lie down.

Hiatus hernia

Sometimes, the hiatus (opening) in the diaphragm is too large, allowing the upper part of the stomach to slip above the diaphragm. The result is that the two parts of the gastro-oesophageal valve are no longer

Hiatus hernia

The hiatus is the small hole in the muscular diaphragm through which the oesophagus passes. If there is a weakness in the hiatus, part of the stomach may slide into the chest – causing a hiatus hernia.

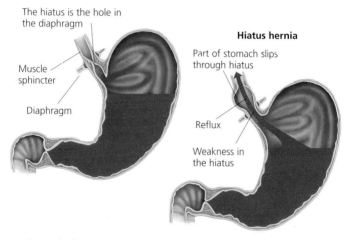

Normal

The hiatus is the hole in the diaphragm

Muscle sphincter

Diaphragm

Hiatus hernia

Part of stomach slips through hiatus

Reflux

Weakness in the hiatus

aligned, thus reducing its strength and allowing reflux of acid into the oesophagus.

Having a hiatus hernia does not always cause symptoms – in fact most people don't get any. What hiatus hernias do is make gastro-oesophageal reflux more likely and this is what causes the symptoms.

No one knows why a hiatus hernia may develop, but they are known to be extremely common (especially in those aged over 65 years) and often they go undetected, causing no trouble throughout a person's whole life.

Consequences of gastro-oesophageal reflux

In most people reflux of acid and pepsin into the oesophagus causes symptoms but does no actual damage. In a small proportion of people, however, there is damage to the lining of the oesophagus in the form of inflammation known as oesophagitis.

Oesophagitis

Although no one knows why some people with reflux get oesophagitis whereas others do not, it is thought to be more likely in tobacco smokers. With appropriate treatment oesophagitis can be healed completely, but if you've had it for a long time there are two more serious consequences: oesophageal strictures and Barrett's oesophagus.

Oesophageal strictures

Long-standing inflammation of the oesophagus can lead to scar formation, which, in turn, can lead to narrowing of the oesophagus, making swallowing difficult. This will require specialist treatment in hospital. The treatment of oesophageal strictures is discussed on page 58.

It is important to emphasise that difficulty swallowing always requires full evaluation by a doctor as soon as possible, and often requires hospital treatment.

Barrett's oesophagus

After many years of exposure to acid, the lining of the oesophagus slowly changes to resemble that of the stomach (with its self-protecting mucus). This condition is named Barrett's oesophagus, after the doctor who first discovered it. In many cases there are no adverse consequences, but it is known to be one of the causes of oesophageal cancer; for this reason, you will probably need to be followed up closely in hospital if the condition is extensive.

How is reflux diagnosed?

Your doctor will normally be able to diagnose gastro-oesophageal reflux from your symptoms without needing to refer you for any tests, especially if, like many people, you've been getting the same symptoms for years.

On the other hand, tests may be needed to confirm the diagnosis or to make sure that you do not have some other condition requiring different treatment if:

- you are over 40 and your symptoms don't respond to treatment

- you have any difficulty swallowing

- you vomit blood or altered blood that looks like coffee grounds.

The most commonly used and most useful test in this context is the upper gastrointestinal endoscopy (see page 29).

A barium X-ray (see page 35) may sometimes be helpful as it will show up any muscle spasm.

In the relatively rare cases where the diagnosis is still not clear from the results of these tests, other possible hospital investigations include measuring the amount of acid in the oesophagus and measuring the pressure within the oesophagus using special probes passed via the nose.

Treatment via lifestyle changes

Treatment of reflux, as with any medical condition, is based first on elimination of the underlying causes. It is most important to change any aspects of your lifestyle that may be making the condition worse, as explained earlier (see page 17):

- If you smoke, make up your mind to stop and do it. Smoking makes heartburn more likely and is bad for your general health.

- Lose weight if necessary – try to take regular exercise as well as making any necessary changes to your diet.

- Keep your alcohol intake to a minimum or cut it out altogether.

- Avoid eating any foods that you know trigger your symptoms. Don't overfill your stomach but rather eat little and often. Always sit down to eat and make a point of eating slowly and chewing your food well.

- Don't wear tight belts or underclothes.

- Don't eat or drink just before going to bed.

- Prop the head end of the bed up by about six inches so that you sleep on a gentle incline – putting telephone directories under the bed head legs works well. You may also find it helpful to sleep on your left side.

- Avoid bending at the waist or stooping immediately after you've eaten.

Making these changes is often all that's necessary for many people, but they don't work for everyone. If your symptoms improve sufficiently so that they trouble you much less than before, you may not need any further treatment.

Medical treatment (from your pharmacist)
Many of the medications available over the counter

Avoiding heartburn at night

If you lie on a horizontal bed it is easier for your stomach contents to leak into the oesophagus and cause heartburn. Sleeping on a bed raised slightly at the head can avoid this.

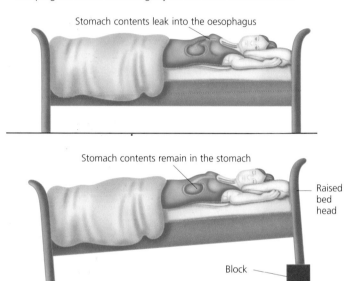

Stomach contents leak into the oesophagus

Stomach contents remain in the stomach

Raised bed head

Block

(from your pharmacist) such as antacids and the H_2-receptor blockers (see pages 20–4), may be all that is needed to control your symptoms. However, your doctor can prescribe more powerful drugs if necessary. These fall broadly into two categories: the proton pump inhibitors and prokinetic drugs. These medicines are available on prescription from your doctor.

Proton pump inhibitors

These are a group of acid-suppressing drugs that have been developed relatively recently, including, for example, omeprazole, lansoprazole and pantoprazole. These are extremely powerful drugs and can be used

How proton pump inhibitors work

These drugs work by preventing the acid-producing cells in the stomach wall from working in the normal way, thereby reducing the amount of acid present in the stomach. They need to be taken on a long-term basis.

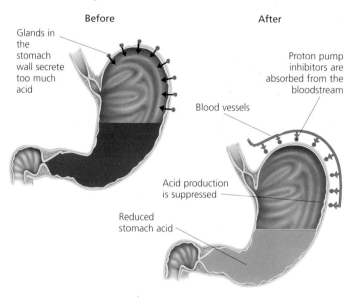

Before

Glands in the stomach wall secrete too much acid

After

Proton pump inhibitors are absorbed from the bloodstream

Blood vessels

Acid production is suppressed

Reduced stomach acid

to treat gastro-oesophageal reflux if your symptoms haven't responded to more simple measures.

They suppress stomach acid only while you are actually taking them, so your symptoms of reflux will come back if you stop. This means that you may have to take them on a long-term basis, rather than as a single 'course' of treatment, in which case side effects become a more crucial factor.

The fact that these drugs are relatively new means that doctors are still building up knowledge about them. They may cause minor side effects, similar to those of the H_2-receptor antagonists, such as drowsiness, headache, rash and possibly confusion in older people. More importantly, proton pump inhibitors are so powerful that they reduce the stomach acid to almost zero. This has two significant effects.

First side effect

One of the functions of stomach acid, as mentioned previously, is that it helps kill any bacteria present in food that you have eaten. Thus, the most common consequence of absence of stomach acid is an increased risk of gastroenteritis. In a normal healthy individual this is not usually a problem (unless they travel abroad, when travellers' diarrhoea may be more common), but very elderly or infirm people may develop severe gastroenteritis.

Second side effect

The second concern about taking proton pump inhibitors long term is that they have been shown to thin the lining of the stomach (a condition known medically as gastric atrophy). Whether this atrophy in individuals taking the drugs long term will turn out to be important is not known, but it is a matter of intense debate among doctors. Currently, proton pump inhibitors are thought to be safe to take long term, although this advice may change in the future. A sensible approach is only to take them long term if absolutely necessary.

Prokinetic drugs

The name 'prokinetic' literally means 'helping movement'. These drugs therefore help the muscles of the stomach wall become more effective at preventing gastro-oesophageal reflux by encouraging the stomach to

How prokinetic drugs work

These drugs do not prevent acid production. Instead they work by helping the muscles of the stomach wall to function more effectively, reducing the likelihood of reflux and helping the stomach to empty more efficiently.

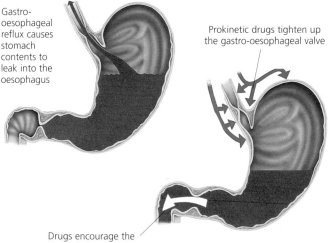

Gastro-oesophageal reflux causes stomach contents to leak into the oesophagus

Prokinetic drugs tighten up the gastro-oesophageal valve

Drugs encourage the stomach to empty

empty more efficiently. In addition, they tighten up the valve at the top of the stomach, which helps to prevent reflux. Both these effects are achieved through the drugs' action on the nerve endings, which control the muscles in the stomach.

As well as playing a role in the treatment of reflux, prokinetic drugs are especially useful for people with an 'anxious' stomach, and are sometimes prescribed for non-ulcer dyspepsia (see page 90), with or without other treatments.

They are usually taken regularly throughout the day and, as with acid-suppressing drugs, they may need to be taken long term. Examples of prokinetic drugs are metoclopramide and domperidone.

Generally these drugs are safe but, because of their prokinetic effects on the intestine, they can cause crampy tummy pain and diarrhoea.

Metoclopramide is not usually given to young women or children because it can cause severe muscle spasms in the face and neck (called a dystonic reaction). This side effect is far less common in men and older women.

Surgery to relieve reflux

Before the advent of potent acid-suppressing drugs, severe gastro-oesophageal reflux was frequently treated by means of surgery. Briefly, the operation has two parts:

1. The surgeon performs an operation to make the hole in the diaphragm smaller with some stitches, thereby correcting any hiatus hernia.

2. He or she tightens the lower oesophageal sphincter using part of the stomach wrapped around itself as a belt.

Originally this operation was a major undertaking requiring several days in hospital and many weeks off work, but now it is usually done as a 'keyhole' procedure and is far less disabling. This is because, instead of working through a large incision, the surgeon operates using endoscopes (viewing tubes) with the help of video cameras, and needs to make only very small cuts through which the instruments are inserted. The result is that recovery time after surgery is much shorter, although the operation may be technically more difficult to perform, especially if the patient is overweight.

With the advent of less arduous operations, and as treatment for gastro-oesophageal reflux may need to be continued over a long period, anti-reflux surgery is once again becoming more popular.

Any operation does, however, carry risks and about 15 per cent of people will have some symptoms afterwards (in particular an inability to belch or vomit), so surgery is usually reserved for those individuals who do not respond to, or cannot take, medical treatment for one reason or another. If surgery is to be considered the surgeon is likely to arrange further tests before going ahead, so as to be sure that the patient would benefit from having it done.

Reflux complications

Complications of gastro-oesophageal reflux usually only affect people who have severe symptoms that have not received treatment, especially if they are elderly, but they can also sometimes be the first sign of the condition. Such complications can be diagnosed only by endoscopy (with or without a biopsy) and/or barium X-ray.

Treatment for oesophagitis

Treatment for oesophagitis is very similar to that for uncomplicated gastro-oesophageal reflux, although for the initial few weeks a proton pump inhibitor (see page 52) is likely to be recommended to ensure that the oesophagitis heals.

Once the oesophagitis has healed, patients are usually given the simplest and least powerful (and therefore least dangerous) treatment that is effective at controlling symptoms long term. In addition to dietary modification and weight loss, occasional simple antacids may be all that is needed. Some patients, however, require more powerful treatment on prescription from their doctor long term, such as H_2-receptor antagonists or even proton pump inhibitors.

Treatment for oesophageal strictures

Scarring and narrowing of the oesophagus, caused by long-standing oesophagitis, may respond to treatment with proton pump inhibitors alone, but if you have any significant difficulty with swallowing, other treatment may also be necessary.

If your oesophagus has become narrowed, it can be stretched during an endoscopy procedure with relative safety, although the problem may recur. This may be done either by passing dilators of gradually increasing size through it, or by inserting a catheter with a deflated balloon into the oesophagus and then inflating the balloon. This stretches the narrowed area and the catheter and balloon can then be removed.

Most doctors recommend that anyone who has had an oesophageal stricture because of reflux should take proton pump inhibitors on a long-term basis (often for the rest of their lives) to help prevent its recurrence. Even with these drugs narrowing can recur, but it usually responds to repeated stretching during a further endoscopy test.

Again it is worth stressing that difficulty swallowing is always important and means that you should see your doctor without delay.

Treatment for Barrett's oesophagus

There is at present no proven effective treatment for this condition, although in the future there may be a role for laser treatment through an endoscope.

Fortunately, the fact that you have it is not likely to interfere with your quality of life or life expectancy.

However, it is known that, over a period of many years, Barrett's oesophagus may develop into an oesophageal cancer; so if your condition is severe and you are young and otherwise fit you are likely to be enrolled in an annual screening programme. This involves having annual endoscopies, looking for signs that a cancer may be about to develop.

If such signs are found, then the only way to prevent cancer developing for certain is an operation to remove the oesophagus, which is an extremely major undertaking. It is for this reason that only those patients fit enough for such an operation are usually offered screening. Depending on how much of the oesophagus needs to be removed, it may be necessary to raise the stomach up higher, or to substitute a piece of colon for the part of the oesophagus that is taken out.

Barrett's oesophagus itself does not cause symptoms, but if you have it you may well need long-term treatment with proton pump inhibitors for severe symptoms caused by gastro-oesophageal reflux.

KEY POINTS

- Heartburn is caused by the reflux of stomach acid into the bottom of the oesophagus

- Drug treatment is aimed at decreasing stomach acidity if simple lifestyle measures are not effective

- In severe cases, reflux of acid can damage the lower end of the oesophagus, necessitating hospital treatment

Peptic ulcers and *H. pylori*

What are peptic ulcers?

They are another major cause of indigestion, although now less common than gastro-oesophageal reflux. Peptic ulcers can occur anywhere in the upper intestinal tract, but they are usually found in the stomach or in the first few inches of the upper intestine, the duodenum.

Medically speaking, an ulcer is a small area of tissue that has lost its upper layers, so that an indentation or sore is created. They are similar in form to mouth ulcers but tend to be deeper and so don't heal as quickly. The 'peptic' part of the name is derived from pepsin, the enzyme that helps break down food, but peptic ulcer disease covers both gastric (stomach) and duodenal ulcers.

Symptoms of peptic ulcers

The predominant symptom caused by peptic ulcers is pain in the central upper abdomen. It is often

How peptic ulcers occur

An ulcer occurs when the mucus layer that protects the stomach or duodenum breaks down and allows acids and enzymes to erode the underlying tissues.

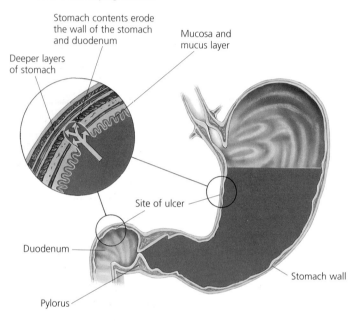

Stomach contents erode the wall of the stomach and duodenum

Deeper layers of stomach

Mucosa and mucus layer

Site of ulcer

Duodenum

Stomach wall

Pylorus

described as a burning pain and can occur at any time, although often it is related to meal times. The symptoms of an ulcer in the stomach or in the duodenum can be identical, but often a duodenal ulcer will cause pain, particularly in the early hours of the morning, that is relieved by a milky drink. A stomach ulcer may cause pain after eating, associated with a feeling of nausea.

One particular feature of the pain is that you can usually pinpoint it very accurately, whereas in other conditions pain tends to be more diffuse. If you have a peptic ulcer your symptoms probably come and go – you may have good periods lasting a few weeks, interspersed with bad periods when you get pain every day. You may well have had symptoms of indigestion on and off for many years.

Causes of peptic ulcers

As mentioned previously, the stomach glands produce a cocktail of acid and pepsin that acts to help digestion of food. The stomach and duodenum protect themselves from acid damage by secreting a layer of protective mucus.

It is when the balance between attack and defence breaks down that a peptic ulcer may develop. There are a number of reasons why this may occur, but the most common cause is a bacterium, the discovery of which has transformed peptic ulcer management.

The helicobacter story

Before the early 1980s peptic ulcers were thought to be caused largely by an individual's lifestyle, although it was acknowledged that other factors might be involved. Peptic ulcers were known to be more common in tobacco smokers and also in those from socially disadvantaged backgrounds. In addition 'stress' was thought to be important, and both patients and doctors often attributed the ulcer to a stressful lifestyle.

With the advent of powerful acid-suppressing drugs – H_2-receptor antagonists in the late 1960s and proton pump inhibitors in the late 1970s – ulcers could often be healed without the need for surgery. However, it was not uncommon for them to recur after treatment, presumably for the same reasons that the ulcer began in the first place.

In the early 1980s two doctors in Australia, Warren and Marshall, working on specimens of stomach tissue,

The *Helicobacter pylori* bacterium

Discovered in the 1980s, this bacterium lives in the mucus lining of the stomach and can cause gastritis. Some affected people will go on to develop a peptic ulcer.

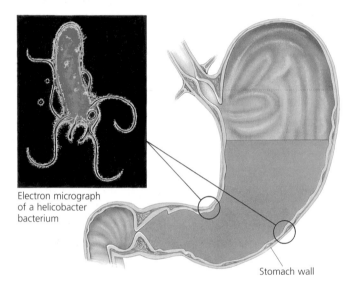

Electron micrograph of a helicobacter bacterium

Stomach wall

discovered a bacterium living in the mucus lining of the lower half of the stomach. The precise role of this bacterium, which they named *Campylobacter pylori*, was unclear. In general, the stomach is sterile, but this bacterium had found a way of concealing itself in the mucus lining where it could not be attacked and destroyed like other bacteria.

Warren and Marshall discovered that, when the infection was present in the stomach, it was always associated with some microscopic inflammation of the lining, called gastritis. At first it was not known whether the infection caused the gastritis or whether the gastritis allowed the infection to occur.

To resolve this issue, Dr Marshall infected himself with the bacterium and tests showed that he did indeed develop gastritis, which disappeared after he successfully eradicated the infection with antibiotics. This proved that it was the infection that caused the gastritis.

More recently the scientific name of the bacterium has been changed to *Helicobacter pylori,* and it has been discovered that a large proportion of the population, possibly as many as 40 per cent, have the infection in their stomachs. Most have no symptoms, but it is now known that a proportion of people – probably around 10 per cent of those infected – will go on to develop a peptic ulcer.

Studies on several thousands of patients with duodenal or gastric ulcers have shown that the vast majority have *H. pylori* infection of the lower stomach and, more importantly, that eradication of the infection with a one-week course of medication results in long-term cure of the ulcer.

How do you become infected?

Helicobacter pylori infection is usually acquired early in life from other members of the family. It can be passed on by close contact and is more common in large families sharing a small house.

You are also more likely to pick up the infection in situations where lots of young adults share a confined space, such as in an army barracks.

Exactly how it is transmitted is not known, but *H. pylori* has been shown to be present in saliva and probably in faeces as well. In most circumstances it is probably impossible to prevent spread of the infection but, as with other intestinal infections, good personal hygiene is important.

As mentioned above, *H. pylori* infection is present in 40 per cent of the entire population. It is known to be more common in those over the age of 65, which may be because the infection was spread more easily under the conditions of the Second World War.

What are the consequences of infection?

Most people infected with *H. pylori* will suffer no symptoms from it for their entire lives. In a proportion (probably in the region of 10 per cent), however, a peptic ulcer will develop.

It is not known why some people develop ulcers whereas others do not, but it probably relates to the age at which the infection was acquired and to the particular type of *H. pylori* with which the person is infected.

The mechanism of ulcer formation is complicated but is probably twofold. *H. pylori* infection in the lower stomach 'fools' the stomach into producing more acid. It also causes thinning of the lining of the stomach, allowing acid to penetrate. Peptic ulcers caused by *H. pylori* infection are otherwise identical to those resulting from other causes, so special tests are usually undertaken to diagnose infection in anyone with a peptic ulcer.

Helicobacter pylori infection without a peptic ulcer does not usually cause any symptoms, although it may play a part in some cases of what is called 'non-ulcer dyspepsia' (see pages 87–92).

In particular *H. pylori* infection does not cause heartburn and gastro-oesophageal reflux. Indeed it is thought that infection may in some way protect against some of the symptoms of reflux and, when *H. pylori* infection is eradicated from people who already have gastro-oesophageal reflux, their symptoms may actually get worse.

This is because, in patients with gastro-oesophageal reflux, those with *H. pylori* infection benefit from a stomach acid-neutralising effect, similar to that of antacids, caused by *H. pylori*. This is different to the effect that *H. pylori* has in patients with a duodenal ulcer, where acid is increased. The reason for these differences is not yet completely understood.

The most controversial area of debate about *H. pylori* infection is whether it can cause stomach cancer. Certainly, infection has not been proved to cause cancer and, more importantly, eradication of the infection has not been shown to reduce the risk of stomach cancer. Eradication of *H. pylori* infection once a stomach cancer has developed has absolutely no effect, but it is certainly effective, and may lead to a complete cure, in patients who have a very rare condition known as lymphoma of the stomach (a tumour of the stomach's blood cells).

Who needs treatment?

The decision as to whether an individual infected with *H. pylori* needs to be treated in order to eradicate the bacterium will be made on the basis of recommendations from the British Society of Gastroenterology and the National Institutes of Health in the USA (see the box on page 68).

How is the infection eradicated?

Helicobacter pylori, unlike the causes of most common infections, is quite difficult to eradicate and you need to take several different drugs at the same time. The reason for this is that the infection resides in a very

Recommendations for the treatment of *Helicobacter pylori*

The British Society of Gastroenterology and the US National Institutes for Health have drawn up guidelines to help doctors decide whether an infected individual needs eradication treatment:

- If you currently have a peptic ulcer, getting rid of *H. pylori* allows it to heal.

- If you have had a peptic ulcer in the past, which was not treated by surgery, eradication prevents it recurring.

- If you do not have and haven't previously had a peptic ulcer, eradication is not necessary if you have gastro-oesophageal reflux, and it may make symptoms worse.

- Eradication of *H. pylori* is not currently recommended in patients with non-ulcer dyspepsia, although this issue is in debate.

- Eradication is not currently thought to be beneficial in preventing stomach cancer, although it is recommended for anyone who has the very rare stomach lymphoma.

- Unless you are in one of the groups of people for whom eradication is thought to be beneficial, you will not need to be tested for *H. pylori* infection.

sheltered environment within the stomach's mucus layer, protected from most drugs. However, over the last 10 years numerous different drug regimes have been developed which, if taken correctly, get rid of the infection in 90 per cent of people who take them.

The most common regimes all consist of three drugs taken together for a period of seven days. Two of the drugs are different antibiotics and the third is a

Eradication of *Helicobacter pylori*

The doctor will prescribe two different types of antibiotics to treat the infection and other drugs to suppress the production of stomach acid.

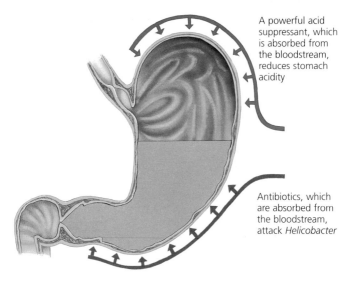

A powerful acid suppressant, which is absorbed from the bloodstream, reduces stomach acidity

Antibiotics, which are absorbed from the bloodstream, attack *Helicobacter*

powerful acid-suppressing drug, usually omeprazole or lansoprazole.

Modern regimes are very safe and cause few problems to those taking them, but some of the anti-biotics can cause nausea and vomiting or diarrhoea (which can be serious in elderly people) and must not be taken with alcohol. It is important to complete the course as prescribed, if possible, because the most common reason why treatment is unsuccessful is that people don't take it properly.

After a course of treatment to eradicate *H. pylori* infection, it is important to check that it has worked by means of one of the *H. pylori* tests described previously (see pages 37–41), usually a urea breath test.

Around one in ten people may need a second course of treatment because the first one has been unsuccessful.

Occasionally, even several courses of treatment fail to eradicate the bacterium and, in this situation, further attempts are usually abandoned in favour of different therapy. It is very unusual for people to become re-infected with the bacterium once it has been successfully eradicated. If symptoms persist after successful eradication of *Helicobacter*, it is because the symptoms are the result of something else.

The future of *H. pylori*

Helicobacter pylori has probably been present in mammals for several thousands of years, and in most seems to cause no ill effects. Although infection undoubtedly causes disease in a few, it may actually have benefits, as yet undiscovered, for the remainder who are infected. This is an area of intense debate among doctors and is one of the reasons why eradication of infection is not recommended routinely for people who do not have ulcers.

It is possible that, in the future, scientists and doctors may discover different 'bad' *H. pylori* and 'good' *H. pylori* and so be able to target only the 'bad' ones for eradication. Along the same lines it is possible that a vaccine could then be developed against 'bad' *H. pylori* and be given to babies, so preventing them acquiring the infection in the first place, and thereby practically eradicating peptic ulcer disease.

KEY POINTS

■ If your doctor suspects a peptic ulcer, further tests of your stomach will be arranged

■ Peptic ulcers occur when the mucus lining of the stomach is damaged by acid

■ The most common cause of peptic ulcer is an infection of the stomach by a bacterium called *Helicobacter pylori*

■ The infection is common, affecting four of ten people; for reasons that are not understood only a minority of people with the infection ever develop an ulcer

■ Peptic ulcers caused by *Helicobacter* can usually be healed with a course of antibiotics to cure the infection

■ Nowadays, surgery is only rarely required to treat complicated ulcers

■ Helicobacter infection by itself, without a peptic ulcer, is treated only in special circumstances

Peptic ulcers – other causes and complications

Anti-arthritis drugs (NSAIDs)

The other main cause of peptic ulcers is the non-steroidal anti-inflammatory drugs (often called simply NSAIDs) used for treatment of arthritis and muscular aches and pains (which include aspirin, indometacin, ibuprofen, diclofenac and naproxen).

Some of these are also used to relieve headaches and period pains, and ibuprofen (sold over the counter under brand names such as Nurofen and Advil) is also found in many cold and flu remedies.

If taken regularly over a long period (to treat rheumatoid arthritis, for example), these drugs may cause ulcers by interfering with the defence system of the duodenum and stomach. Occasional use of the drugs rarely has the same effect, but they may make symptoms worse if an ulcer already exists.

NSAIDs and stomach ulcers

Some anti-arthritis drugs (NSAIDs) can interfere with the digestive system.

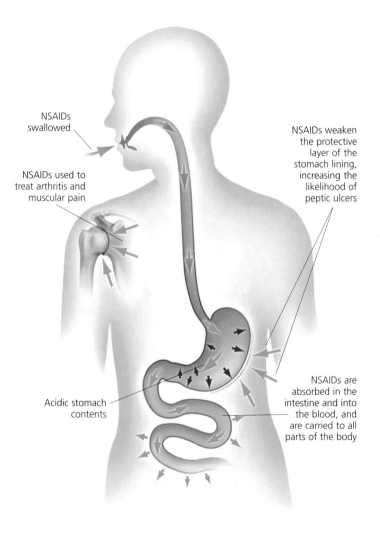

NSAIDs swallowed

NSAIDs used to treat arthritis and muscular pain

Acidic stomach contents

NSAIDs weaken the protective layer of the stomach lining, increasing the likelihood of peptic ulcers

NSAIDs are absorbed in the intestine and into the blood, and are carried to all parts of the body

These drugs exert their anti-inflammatory effect within the body by reducing the production of chemicals called prostaglandins. If you injure yourself or get an infected cut, it becomes hot, red and painful. This is the result of prostaglandins, chemicals released from damaged cells around the injury. In most parts of the body (for example, inside the joints of people with arthritic conditions) where prostaglandins make inflammation worse.

NSAIDs are very effective. In the stomach, however, prostaglandins are a very important part of the mucus layer defence system, and general, widely acting NSAIDs also decrease these prostaglandins, weakening the stomach's defence and allowing peptic ulcers to develop in some people.

Newer NSAIDs (known as cyclo-oxygenase 2 or COX-2 inhibitors) have been developed. These reduce prostaglandin production in the rest of the body without affecting production in the stomach. COX-2 inhibitors include celecoxib, valdecoxib, paracoxib and etoricoxib. COX-2 inhibitors have fewer gastrointestinal side effects than traditional NSAIDs.

Unfortunately they may also have severe side effects in the heart and circulatory system in certain susceptible patients, so you should always discuss such treatments with your doctor very carefully.

Other causes of pepic ulcers

Peptic ulcers very occasionally occur in people who do not have *Helicobacter pylori* infection and who are not on NSAIDs. These ulcers, although they usually respond well to treatment, often remain unexplained.

Very rarely peptic ulcers may be caused by other conditions, usually diagnosed only in hospital.

Examples are:

- Crohn's disease (a condition that can affect any part of the intestine)

- Zollinger–Ellison syndrome (named after the doctors who first discovered it, a condition in which the stomach produces too much acid as a result of a hormone imbalance)

- lymphoma (a tumour of the blood cells within the stomach wall).

Smoking also makes people more likely to have peptic ulcers. It does this by increasing the risk in people carrying the helicobacter infection, and possibly also increasing the risk in patients taking NSAIDs. Smoking also significantly impairs ulcer healing. Anyone who has or has had an ulcer and smokes is always advised to stop.

Complications of peptic ulcers

In most cases, peptic ulcers cause rather unpleasant symptoms but nothing more serious. There are, however, three potentially serious complications:

- bleeding

- perforation

- pyloric stenosis.

Although it is also the case that people with stomach cancer are sometimes found to have a gastric ulcer, there is no real evidence that 'ordinary', benign stomach ulcers can become cancerous.

Bleeding

Occasionally a peptic ulcer can 'burrow' into one of the arteries of the stomach or duodenum wall and cause bleeding. This can be very severe, and blood may then be vomited up or pass through the intestine and appear in the motions. Vomit that contains old blood actually looks like coffee grounds because of the way the blood changes its appearance after being in contact with stomach acid. Similarly, once blood has travelled through the intestine it appears jet black and tarry. This is always important and, whether you have indigestion or not, you should always see your doctor straightaway after vomiting blood or passing jet-black tarry motions.

Perforation

Occasionally, a peptic ulcer may erode completely through the stomach or duodenum wall so that

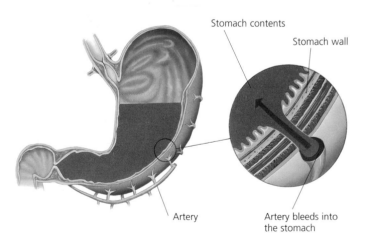

Stomach contents

Stomach wall

Artery

Artery bleeds into the stomach

Bleeding: occasionally a peptic ulcer can burrow into an artery.

stomach acid gets into the abdominal cavity, causing peritonitis (inflammation of the abdominal cavity). If there is any leakage of stomach contents into the abdomen, the person experiences severe pain and infection may develop.

This usually happens out of the blue to someone who has been suffering from indigestion and, as it can be fatal without treatment, emergency surgery will be needed immediately to repair the hole.

Pyloric stenosis

This is the medical name for a condition in which the pylorus – the valve at the bottom of the stomach – becomes narrowed and so doesn't work properly. Repeated ulceration, over a period of several months or years, at the junction between the stomach and

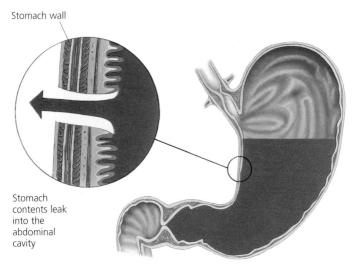

Stomach wall

Stomach contents leak into the abdominal cavity

Perforation: occasionally a peptic ulcer may erode through the stomach wall, allowing the stomach contents to leak.

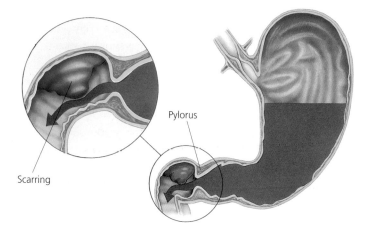

Pyloric stenosis: the valve at the bottom of the stomach becomes narrowed and doesn't work properly. Repeated ulceration causes scarring which obstructs normal stomach emptying.

duodenum can cause a severe scar so tight that it does not allow food and liquid to leave the stomach.

Unlike ordinary tissue, an area that is scarred is not flexible and has a tendency to shrink over time. Sometimes pyloric stenosis may be caused by swelling around an ulcer, but the swelling will subside if the person is given acid-suppressing drug treatment.

The condition may develop in someone who has had indigestion on and off for years, and the main symptoms are recurrent vomiting and a feeling of fullness. It can usually be treated successfully with drugs, but occasionally an operation to enlarge the opening may be necessary if the narrowing is very severe.

Stomach cancer

Very occasionally, a person with a stomach ulcer (though not a duodenal ulcer) may be found to have stomach cancer (see page 93). For this reason, whenever a stomach ulcer is diagnosed specimens are usually taken from it to be examined under the microscope for evidence of cancer cells.

If you have a stomach ulcer, normally you will be followed up closely with regular hospital checks to make sure that your ulcer is healing with treatment. Treatment is otherwise similar to that for duodenal ulcers – that is, antibiotics and acid-suppressing drugs (see page 81).

KEY POINTS

- Anti-inflammatory drugs and aspirin can cause peptic ulcers by damaging the stomach's lining

- If you develop indigestion while taking one of these treatments, you should consult your doctor

- If you experience symptoms such as vomiting or passing blood in the motions, recurrent vomiting or severe abdominal pain, consult your doctor immediately

Treating a peptic ulcer

Confirming the diagnosis

Even though your doctor may be fairly certain from your symptoms that you have a peptic ulcer, he or she will usually arrange for you to have further tests to confirm the diagnosis.

The most reliable of those currently available is the upper gastrointestinal endoscopy, often known simply as endoscopy. This has largely replaced barium X-ray tests (although these are still occasionally required).

Helicobacter pylori infection can also be diagnosed at the time of an endoscopy test (in addition to other means). For details of these tests, see pages 37–41.

Medical treatment for ulcers

Treatment of peptic ulcers has been revolutionised over the last decade or so by the advent of newer ulcer-healing drugs, in addition to the discovery that eradication of *Helicobacter pylori* infection is often all that is required.

Although lifestyle changes such as giving up smoking are important and will help, they are unlikely to be successful alone in treating peptic ulcers (unlike in the case of gastro-oesophageal reflux).

Treatment of peptic ulcers varies slightly depending on whether you are taking non-steroidal anti-inflammatory drugs at the time your ulcer is diagnosed.

Ulcers caused by *Helicobacter pylori* infection

Before the discovery of *Helicobacter pylori* (*H. pylori*), patients with peptic ulcers were treated with acid-suppressing drugs such as H_2-receptor antagonists or proton pump inhibitors. These drugs are identical to the ones used to treat gastro-oesophageal reflux, discussed on pages 51–6.

When given for eight weeks these drugs are very effective at healing the ulcer, but they have no effect on the underlying cause, that is, *H. pylori* infection. This means that the ulcer may come back in the future, and in years gone by patients required intermittent treatment for peptic ulcers for many years.

Now it is known that if you have a peptic ulcer caused by *H. pylori* then eradication of the bacterium is all that is required. This will not only allow the ulcer to heal, but also prevent it coming back.

Acid-suppressing drugs are not usually necessary after a course of eradication treatment unless the ulcer caused some internal bleeding, in which case doctors like to give eight weeks of acid-suppressing treatment as a 'belt and braces' approach.

Modern treatments for *H. pylori* infection consist of three drugs taken together for a week. These are two antibiotics taken with a proton pump inhibitor. Treatment of *H. pylori* infection is described in more detail on pages 67–70.

Ulcers caused by taking non-steroidal anti-inflammatory drugs

As discussed previously, patients taking a non-steroidal anti-inflammatory drug (NSAID) may get peptic ulcers as a result of the drugs themselves. These patients may also have *H. pylori* infection but usually the NSAIDs are the most important factor.

If possible, the NSAID treatment should be stopped or substituted for a less damaging treatment such as paracetamol or possibly one of the newer, potentially safer NSAIDs.

The ulcer itself is treated in traditional fashion with an eight-week course of a proton pump inhibitor, one of the more powerful acid-suppressing drugs. Nowadays less powerful acid-suppressing drugs, the H_2-receptor antagonists such as cimetidine or ranitidine, are not considered sufficient for healing the ulcer.

If you are able to stop taking the NSAIDs then no further treatment may be required. If you cannot stop your anti-inflammatory treatment, however, you may also be prescribed a proton pump inhibitor to take long term to prevent your ulcer coming back. Proton pump inhibitors are currently regarded as the best treatment to prevent the damage caused by NSAIDs. The current evidence is that H_2-receptor antagonists are not sufficient for this purpose.

Another drug that is used is misoprostol. Instead of suppressing the stomach's acid, misoprostol prevents ulcers in patients by helping to boost the defences of the stomach and duodenum against the damaging effect of NSAIDs. It is chemically similar to the natural prostaglandin chemicals found in the stomach lining, which are inhibited by NSAIDs.

Although misoprostol is safe it does cause diarrhoea in some people, which limits its usefulness. Misoprostol is not given to premenopausal women who are capable of conceiving children because it causes miscarriages.

Ulcers caused by NSAIDs with *H. pylori* infection

At the moment doctors do not agree on whether *H. pylori* infection should be treated in patients with ulcers caused by NSAIDs.

Some doctors feel that the infection should always be eradicated if an ulcer is present, whether or not patients have taken NSAIDs.

Recent evidence, however, shows that eradicating the infection may make no difference or, worse, make ulcers more difficult to heal.

The current advice is that the *H. pylori* infection need not be eradicated in these cases, although this advice may change in the future.

Surgical treatment for ulcers

Before newer treatments became available surgery was commonly recommended for people with peptic ulcers. These days it is required only to treat some complications of ulcers and, very occasionally, when ulcers do not respond to treatment.

There are many different operations available but the general aim of surgical treatment is to reduce the acid secretion of the stomach glands by cutting the nerves that supply the stomach (a procedure known as a vagotomy). Another consequence of a vagotomy is that the stomach cannot empty properly afterwards so, in addition, the surgeon performs an operation on the stomach itself to correct this.

Conclusion

Peptic ulcers are reasonably common and, if your doctor suspects that this is the cause of your symptoms, the best way to confirm the diagnosis is for you to have an endoscopy.

The most common cause of a peptic ulcer is infection with *Helicobacter pylori*, and eradication of this infection with antibiotics is often all that is required to heal the ulcer. The other main cause of peptic ulcers is treatment with NSAIDs.

Peptic ulcers can nearly always be healed with drugs and surgery is only very rarely necessary. One complication of peptic ulcers is bleeding, so you should consult your doctor immediately if you vomit blood or pass black, tarry motions.

KEY POINTS

- Peptic ulcers can be healed by a course of acid-suppressing drug treatment

- Once a peptic ulcer is diagnosed, it is important to treat the underlying cause

- Anti-inflammatory drug treatment should be stopped until the ulcer is healed

- If *H. pylori* infection is present, it will be eradicated with antibiotics to prevent the ulcer recurring

- Surgery is reserved for ulcers that do not heal with drug treatment and for complicated ulcers

Non-ulcer dyspepsia

What are the symptoms?

Your doctor is likely to diagnose this condition if you have indigestion-type symptoms but tests show that your stomach and duodenum are normal – that is, there is no evidence of ulceration or gastro-oesophageal reflux.

There is no diagnostic test for non-ulcer dyspepsia so before it is diagnosed other likely conditions causing similar symptoms usually need to be ruled out, either by a physical examination or by other tests. Conditions that may masquerade as non-ulcer dyspepsia are shown in the box on page 88.

The main symptoms of non-ulcer dyspepsia are burning and aching in the upper abdomen, which is usually related in some way to eating (food makes it either better or worse), and occasionally nausea.

In addition many people suffer from what is often called a 'nervous stomach': their symptoms are often worse at times of stress. It is not known what causes

What else might the pain be?

There is no specific test for non-ulcer dyspepsia, so before making a firm diagnosis your doctor needs to rule out some other conditions that have similar symptoms.

- Gallstones
  Stones that may vary in size from that of small pieces of gravel up to 2–3 centimetres in diameter, and consist of cholesterol and the breakdown products of red blood cells. They form in the gallbladder and irritate its lining, especially after eating fatty foods, when the gallbladder contracts and causes pain. Sometimes they may get stuck in the bile duct and cause jaundice.

- Irritable bowel syndrome (IBS)
  This is a very common condition that is associated with muscle spasm within the walls of the intestines. The cause is unknown but the symptoms often seem to be related to stress in many people.

- Muscle pain
  Pain arising from the lower ribs and muscles of the abdominal wall.

non-ulcer dyspepsia but there are likely to be many factors. One theory is that, for some reason, the stomachs of people with this condition are far more sensitive to stimuli such as normal stomach acid and certain food-stuffs. Another theory suggests that, particularly in people with a 'nervous stomach', the muscles of the stomach wall become especially tense at times of stress, so making the symptoms worse.

From a strictly medical point of view, non-ulcer dyspepsia is never a serious condition, but it can be a severe nuisance. It is important to be sure that it really is the true cause of a person's symptoms. In particular, it very rarely causes weight loss so, if you have indigestion and are losing weight at the same time, your doctor needs to look for other, possibly more serious, causes for your symptoms. If you are taking non-steroidal anti-inflammatory drugs (NSAIDs), your doctor also needs to rule out peptic ulceration before diagnosing non-ulcer dyspepsia.

Treatment
Self-help measures

The most important step is to understand the condition and realise that your symptoms are not the result of something more serious. The next step is to try to alter any aspect of your lifestyle that is making your symptoms worse.

Generally speaking, the most important changes that you can make towards achieving a healthier way of living are to:

- stop smoking

- lose weight if necessary

- make sure that you are eating the right kind of diet.

The most common dietary culprits when it comes to making this kind of indigestion worse are fatty or fried foods, hot and spicy foods, certain vegetables such as onions and tomatoes, and occasionally caffeine in the form of tea, coffee and cola-type drinks. If you find that any of these things upset you, cut them out.

Make a point of increasing your daily intake of high-fibre foods. This not only often helps to relieve symptoms of non-ulcer dyspepsia but also helps to protect you against many other conditions, such as heart disease, high blood pressure and bowel cancer. Suitable fibre is found in fruit and vegetables, high-fibre breakfast cereals and whole-grain bread.

Medical treatment

There is no true drug 'panacea' for non-ulcer dyspepsia. Certain drugs are effective but they are usually prescribed only for people whose symptoms are still intolerable even though they have followed all the lifestyle advice given above.

Unlike the acid-related disorders of peptic ulcer and gastro-oesophageal reflux, non-ulcer dyspepsia does not usually respond to treatment with antacid medication. The drugs that are most effective are usually those that alter the way the stomach empties itself. Examples of these 'prokinetic' drugs, which are available only on prescription, are domperidone and metoclopramide (see page 54). Tablets are taken half an hour before meals to help the stomach muscles coordinate correctly, thus reducing symptoms of tension in the stomach wall and nausea.

Treatment with these drugs often has to be continued for several months, so knowing about possible side effects is important. As these drugs have an effect on the movement not only of the stomach but also of the intestine, they sometimes cause crampy lower abdominal pain and diarrhoea.

Generally they are safe, but more severe side effects can occur – in particular metoclopramide is not usually given to young women and children because it can cause neck and face muscle spasms, known as a dystonic reaction (this side effect is much less common in men and older women).

Conclusion

Non-ulcer dyspepsia is very common and, although often uncomfortable, is not serious. Symptoms of upper abdominal discomfort and nausea can often be easily controlled by lifestyle changes such as stress reduction, stopping smoking, weight loss and healthier eating.

A minority of people who still have severe symptoms despite lifestyle changes may need treatment with prokinetic drugs. Non-ulcer dyspepsia should not be confused with more serious conditions requiring different treatment.

If you are losing weight (or have done so without trying) or if you are taking NSAIDs and develop new indigestion symptoms, you should see your doctor.

KEY POINTS

- Non-ulcer dyspepsia is one of the most common causes of indigestion and is never serious

- Treatment is based on understanding the condition and avoiding certain foods that make it worse

Stomach cancer

What is cancer?

A lump of human tissue the size of a sugar cube may contain a thousand million cells. These are the minute building blocks from which our bodies are made, visible only down the microscope. It is quite amazing that the billions of cells in a human body normally function in perfect harmony, every cell knowing its place and doing the job that it was designed to do. Most cells have a finite lifespan: millions of new ones are produced every day to replace those lost through old age or wear and tear.

New cells are produced when existing cells divide into two. Except in children, who are growing, there is normally a perfect balance between the numbers of the cells that are dying and those that are dividing. Normally exactly the right amounts of new cells are produced to replace those that are being lost. The control mechanisms involved are exceedingly complex. Loss of control can lead to an excess of cells, resulting in a tumour.

However, it is important to realise that only a very small minority of tumours are cancerous. Most tumours

How a tumour forms

A cancerous tumour begins as a single cell. If it is not destroyed by the body's immune system, it will double into two cells, which in turn divide into four and so on.

Cancerous cell

First doubling

Second doubling

are localised accumulations of normal or fairly normal cells and are benign. A wart is a common example.

The development of a cancer (malignant tumour) involves a change in the quality of the cells as well as an increase in quantity: they change in both appearance and behaviour. They become more aggressive, destructive and independent of normal cells. They acquire the ability to infiltrate and invade the surrounding tissues.

In some instances the cells may also invade lymphatic and blood vessels and thus spread away from the 'primary' growth to other places. In time these cells may cause the development of secondary growths, known as 'metastases', in the lymph glands and other organs such as lungs, liver and bones.

Stomach cancer

Stomach cancer, although far less common than other causes of indigestion, is an extremely serious condition that must be diagnosed early on if treatment is to be effective. The cancer develops in cells lining the stomach, called glandular cells.

If untreated, it can then spread to involve the whole thickness of the stomach and, via the bloodstream, the liver. This process can occur relatively quickly, which is

How cancer spreads

Cancerous tumours can spread to distant sites in the body by a process called metastasis. In metastasis the cancerous cell separates from a malignant tumour and travels to a new location in the blood or lymph.

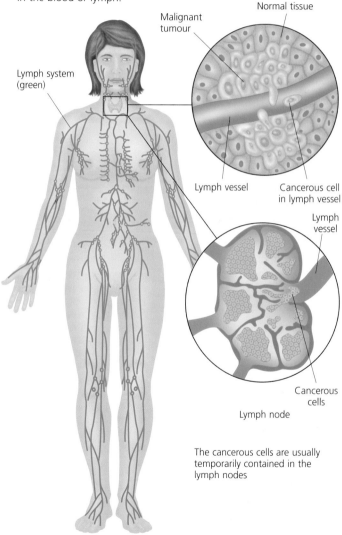

Normal tissue

Malignant tumour

Lymph system (green)

Lymph vessel

Cancerous cell in lymph vessel

Lymph vessel

Cancerous cells

Lymph node

The cancerous cells are usually temporarily contained in the lymph nodes

why the condition is so difficult to treat unless picked up early on.

Although the person concerned may consult their doctor because of a burning upper abdominal pain (similar to peptic ulcer), it usually causes more of an ache and they may often be off their food and feel very full after even quite small meals. As a result of the loss of appetite, weight loss is common. The combination of these symptoms should always be taken seriously and should always be assessed by a doctor.

What causes stomach cancer?

The actual cause of stomach cancer is not known and it may be the result of a variety of factors. There are no proven genetic links, and it is more likely that stomach cancer is caused by environmental factors. Certainly, stomach cancer is more common in some countries than others – it is far more common in the Far East than in Europe and this may be caused by, among other things, a difference in diet between the two populations. It is known that the descendants of Japanese emigrants to the west have the same incidence of stomach cancer as westerners, supporting the influence of environment over genetics.

It is clear that *Helicobacter pylori* infection plays a central role in causing stomach cancer. However, it is not known whether eradication of the infection would actually lead to a decreased risk of stomach cancer. Currently, the medical authorities in the UK and the USA do not recommend treatment for this purpose, although the position may change in the future.

Fortunately, the incidence of stomach cancer in Europe and the west is decreasing, although again this is unexplained. Stomach cancer is usually a disease of late middle-aged and elderly people, although it may occur rarely in people under 40.

How is it diagnosed?

This normally happens when an endoscopy test is done, although it may be diagnosed with a barium X-ray. As effective treatment is available only if the disease is caught early, anyone with indigestion who also has what doctors call the 'sinister' symptoms of lack of appetite and weight loss will need to be thoroughly investigated.

As stomach cancer is more common in those aged over 40, full investigation is usually a good idea in anyone over this age who has indigestion for the first time, with or without sinister symptoms.

Is there a cure?

The only curative treatment is an operation to remove the stomach and all of the cancer. It is most effective when the disease is in its early stages, hence the need for an early diagnosis and the importance of taking seriously such symptoms as weight loss and feeling full after eating a small amount.

Sometimes, the surgeon may be able to leave part of the stomach in place; otherwise, food will have to go directly from the oesophagus to the small intestine after the operation. This means that the person will then have to eat little and often, and may well need to take food supplements because digestion is impaired.

If the cancer is small and the surgeon can remove it all then the chance of long-term cure is very good, but unfortunately the disease is often advanced at the time of diagnosis and surgery is not possible.

Currently, if surgery is not possible or is unsuccessful, then other forms of treatment are unlikely to result in cure. These other forms of treatment, such as chemotherapy and laser therapy, do, however, have a very valuable role in controlling uncomfortable symptoms, and may prolong life considerably.

Conclusion

As treatment for advanced stomach cancer is often unsatisfactory, it is very important to make the diagnosis early on in the course of the disease.

Weight loss, loss of appetite and new symptoms in someone aged over 40 may be a sign of early stomach cancer and should always be assessed by a doctor. In the future, when the cause of the disease is better understood, the emphasis will be placed more on prevention of stomach cancer, but currently efforts are continually being made to improve non-surgical treatments, such as chemotherapy.

KEY POINTS

- Stomach cancer is very rare in people under the age of 40

- New symptoms after the age of 40, or sinister symptoms such as weight loss and loss of appetite, should always be discussed with a doctor

- Stomach cancer can be diagnosed only using hospital-based tests

Points to remember

The aim of this booklet is to help you to understand the causes of indigestion so that you have confidence to be able to decide on the most appropriate course of action.

The most important question when considering your own symptoms is whether an expert opinion is required to rule out a serious condition that requires further investigation. Throughout the booklet we have tried to highlight those symptoms that are 'sinister' and that always require medical advice from the outset:

- Unexplained weight loss

- Loss of appetite

- Difficulty swallowing

- Vomiting blood or material that looks like coffee grounds

- Passing altered blood in the motions – this makes your stools look 'tarry'

- Indigestion when taking non-steroidal anti-inflammatory drugs (NSAIDs).

Indigestion without these sinister symptoms can be treated sensibly at home in the first instance with lifestyle measures:

- lose some weight

- stop smoking

- change your diet.

If these measures are not effective, the next step is to try antacids. The easiest and best source of initial advice about antacids is your local pharmacist, who will have a full knowledge about the causes, and treatment, of indigestion.

If these simple measures provide symptomatic relief then it may not be necessary to see your doctor. However, if symptoms remain after treating yourself for two weeks, or if you are over 40 and develop symptoms for the first time, then it is always wise to seek medical advice.

Useful addresses

Where can I find out more?

We have included the following organisations because, on preliminary investigation, they may be of use to the reader. However, we do not have first-hand experience of each organisation and so cannot guarantee the organisation's integrity. The reader must therefore exercise his or her own discretion and judgement when making further enquiries.

Benefits Enquiry Line

Tel: 0800 882200
Minicom: 0800 243355
Website: www.dwp.gov.uk
N. Ireland: 0800 220674
Minicom: 0800 243789

Government agency giving information and advice on sickness and disability benefits for people with disabilities and their carers.

Citizens Advice Bureaux

Myddleton House, 115–123 Pentonville Road
London N1 9LZ
Tel: 020 7833 2181 (admin only)
Website: www.adviceguide.org.uk

HQ of national charity offering a wide variety of
practical, financial and legal advice. Network of local
charities throughout the UK listed in phone books and
in *Yellow Pages* under 'C'.

CORE (Digestive Disorders Foundation)

3 St Andrew's Place, Regents Park
London NW1 4LB
Tel: 020 7486 0341
Fax: 020 7224 2012
Email: info@corecharity.org.uk
Website: www.corecharity.org.uk

Provides a range of leaflets about the cause, symptoms
and treatment of digestive disorders. Please send an
SAE when requesting information. Medical advice not
available.

IBS Network – The Irritable Bowel Syndrome Network

Unit 5, 53 Mowbray Street
Sheffield S3 8EN
Tel: 0114 272 3253 (Mon–Fri 6–8pm, Sat 10am–12
noon)
Fax: 0114 261 0112
Email: info@ibsnetwork.org.uk
Website: www.ibsnetwork.org.uk

Publishes factsheets and quarterly newsletter and coordinates local self-help groups that offer a befriending scheme giving support to fellow sufferers. Advice helpline staffed by IBS specialist nurses. An SAE must accompany written enquiries.

NHS Direct
Tel: 0845 4647 (24 hours, 365 days a year)
Textphone: 0845 606 4647
Website: www.nhsdirect.nhs.uk
NHS Scotland: 0800 224488

Offers confidential healthcare advice, information and referral service. A good first port of call for any health advice.

NHS Smoking Helpline
Tel: 0800 169 0169 (7am–11pm, 365 days a year)
Pregnancy smoking helpline: 0800 169 9169
(12 noon–9pm, 365 days a year)
Website: www.givingupsmoking.co.uk
N. Ireland: 0800 858585 (12 noon–11pm, 365 days a year)
Scotland: 0800 84484 (12 noon–12 midnight, 365 days a year)
Wales: 0800 085 2219

Have advice, help and encouragement on giving up smoking. Specialist advisers available to offer on-going support to those who genuinely are trying to give up smoking. Can refer to local branches.

National Institute for Health and Clinical Excellence (NICE)

MidCity Place, 71 High Holborn
London WC1V 6NA
Tel: 020 7067 5800
Fax: 020 7067 5801
Email: nice@nice.org.uk
Website: www.nice.org.uk

Provides national guidance on the promotion of good health and the prevention and treatment of ill-health. Patient information leaflets are available for each piece of guidance issued.

Prodigy Website

Sowerby Centre for Health Informatics at Newcastle (SCHIN), Bede House, All Saints Business Centre
Newcastle upon Tyne NE1 2ES
Tel: 0191 243 6100
Fax: 0191 243 6101
Email: prodigy-enquiries@schin.co.uk
Website: www.prodigy.nhs.uk

A website mainly for GPs giving information for patients listed by disease plus named self-help organisations.

Quit (Smoking Quitlines)

211 Old Street
London EC1V 9NR
Helpline: 0800 00 200 (9am–9pm, 365 days a year)
Tel: 020 7251 1551
Fax: 020 7251 1661
Email: info@quit.org.uk
Website: www.quit.org.uk

Offers individual advice on giving up smoking in English and Asian languages. Talks to schools on smoking and can refer to local support groups. Runs training courses for professionals.

The internet as a further source of information

After reading this book, you may feel that you would like further information on the subject. The internet is of course an excellent place to look and there are many websites with useful information about medical disorders, related charities and support groups.

For those who do not have a computer at home some bars and cafes offer facilities for accessing the internet. These are listed in the *Yellow Pages* under 'Internet Bars and Cafes' and 'Internet Providers'. Your local library offers a similar facility and has staff to help you find the information that you need.

It should always be remembered, however, that the internet is unregulated and anyone is free to set up a website and add information to it. Many websites offer impartial advice and information that has been compiled and checked by qualified medical professionals. Some, on the other hand, are run by commercial organisations with the purpose of promoting their own products. Others still are run by pressure groups, some of which will provide carefully assessed and accurate information whereas others may be suggesting medications or treatments that are not supported by the medical and scientific community.

Unless you know the address of the website you want to visit – for example, www.familydoctor.co.uk – you may find the following guidelines useful when searching the internet for information.

Search engines and other searchable sites

Google (www.google.co.uk) is the most popular search engine used in the UK, followed by Yahoo! (http://uk.yahoo.com) and MSN (www.msn.co.uk). Also popular are the search engines provided by Internet Service Providers such as Tiscali and other sites such as the BBC site (www.bbc.co.uk).

In addition to the search engines that index the whole web, there are also medical sites with search facilities, which act almost like mini-search engines, but cover only medical topics or even a particular area of medicine. Again, it is wise to look at who is responsible for compiling the information offered to ensure that it is impartial and medically accurate. The NHS Direct site (www.nhsdirect.nhs.uk) is an example of a searchable medical site.

Links to many British medical charities can be found at the Association of Medical Research Charities' website (www.amrc.org.uk) and at Charity Choice (www.charitychoice.co.uk).

Search phrases

Be specific when entering a search phrase. Searching for information on 'cancer' will return results for many different types of cancer as well as on cancer in general. You may even find sites offering astrological information. More useful results will be returned by using search phrases such as 'lung cancer' and 'treatments for lung cancer'. Both Google and Yahoo! offer an advanced search option that includes the ability to search for the exact phrase, enclosing the search phrase in quotes, that is, 'treatments for lung cancer' will have the same effect. Limiting a search to an exact phrase reduces the number of results returned but it is best to refine a search to an exact match only if you are not getting useful results with a normal search. Adding 'UK' to your search term will bring up mainly British sites, so a good phrase might be 'lung cancer' UK (don't include UK within the quotes).

Always remember the internet is international and unregulated. It holds a wealth of valuable information but individual sites may be biased, out of date or just plain wrong. Family Doctor Publications accepts no responsibility for the content of links published in this series.

Index

Your pages

We have included the following pages because they may help you manage your illness or condition and its treatment.

Before an appointment with a health professional, it can be useful to write down a short list of questions of things that you do not understand, so that you can make sure that you do not forget anything.

Some of the sections may not be relevant to your circumstances.

We are always pleased to receive constructive criticism or suggestions about how to improve the books. You can contact us at:

Email: familydoctor@btinternet.com
Letter: Family Doctor Publications
          PO Box 4664
          Poole
          BH15 1NN

Thank you

Health-care contact details

Name:

Job title:

Place of work:

Tel:

Name:

Job title:

Place of work:

Tel:

Name:

Job title:

Place of work:

Tel:

Name:

Job title:

Place of work:

Tel:

Significant past health events – illnesses/operations/investigations/treatments

Event	Month	Year	Age (at time)

Appointments for health care

Name:

Place:

Date:

Time:

Tel:

Name:

Place:

Date:

Time:

Tel:

Name:

Place:

Date:

Time:

Tel:

Name:

Place:

Date:

Time:

Tel:

Appointments for health care

Name:

Place:

Date:

Time:

Tel:

Name:

Place:

Date:

Time:

Tel:

Name:

Place:

Date:

Time:

Tel:

Name:

Place:

Date:

Time:

Tel:

Current medication(s) prescribed by your doctor

Medicine name:

Purpose:

Frequency & dose:

Start date:

End date:

Medicine name:

Purpose:

Frequency & dose:

Start date:

End date:

Medicine name:

Purpose:

Frequency & dose:

Start date:

End date:

Medicine name:

Purpose:

Frequency & dose:

Start date:

End date:

Other medicines/supplements you are taking, not prescribed by your doctor

Medicine/treatment:

Purpose:

Frequency & dose:

Start date:

End date:

Medicine/treatment:

Purpose:

Frequency & dose:

Start date:

End date:

Medicine/treatment:

Purpose:

Frequency & dose:

Start date:

End date:

Medicine/treatment:

Purpose:

Frequency & dose:

Start date:

End date:

Questions to ask at appointments

(Note: do bear in mind that doctors work under great time pressure, so long lists may not be helpful for either of you)

Questions to ask at appointments

(Note: do bear in mind that doctors work under great time pressure, so long lists may not be helpful for either of you)

Notes